Yoga
to Ease Anxiety

Practices and Perspectives To Help You Enjoy Life Again

Amy Vaughn M.A., RYT

May you find peace and joy!

Amy Vaughn

ISBN:1496140133
ISBN-13:978-1496140135

DEDICATION

For you, really.

CONTENTS

ACKNOWLEDGMENTS

This book would not have been possible without the support and guidance of many important people. Firstly, I want to thank those I took with me through the wringer for being there when I needed you most. There is no way to fully express my gratitude to Rich and Ben Bruso for giving me a reason to live. My appreciation for my parents, Jay and Sharon Vaughn, is endless for their support and understanding and for providing a safe haven for Ben when I wasn't able to be the parent he needed.

To my teachers, Macaela Cashman, Gary Giangregorio, Marcia Galleher, Georg Feuerstein, and Priscilla Potter, you have my deepest gratitude for lighting my path when I was in darkness.

And finally, to everyone on whom I forced a premature copy of this book—Sorry! Thank you each for your patience and insights.

INTRODUCTION

Yoga means different things to different people. At its broadest, yoga refers to the mystical paths of Hinduism, Jainism, and Buddhism. At its most narrow, yoga is an exercise class at the gym. For those of us with anxiety, the most useful definition of yoga may be from Patanjali, who wrote in or around the second century CE that "Yoga is the stilling of the fluctuations of the mind." Doesn't that sound great right about now? I'm going to say it again. "Yoga is the stilling of the fluctuations of the mind."

I've struggled with anxiety all my life. Yoga has helped me through some of my hardest times and continues to help me keep it together today. This book is a personal spin on a problem that everyone experiences in their own personal way. I don't expect every idea to be helpful to every reader, but I do hope that every reader can find something helpful. I've tried to write conversationally, while getting right to the point. I use the pronouns "we" and "our" a lot because I live by what I've written here.

Two major streams of my life have come together in the creation of this book. The longest running of which is my experience with generalized anxiety and the free-floating fear, self-doubt, perfectionism, achievement and recognition needs, worrying, scripting, obsessing, and depression that came with it. I was anxious even as a child and in adulthood my anxiety fully bloomed into panic disorder, obsessive-compulsive habits, and finally agoraphobia, which means I was so afraid of being afraid that I cut myself off from the world as much as I possibly could. I thought of dying often.

The other stream feeding this river is my academic background. In college, I studied religion and psychology. In graduate school, I was able to delve deeply into mysticism. More recently, I completed an 800 hour course of study in the history and philosophy of yoga through Traditional Yoga Studies under Georg and Brenda Feuerstein. I was incredibly fortunate to study under Georg for a year before he passed on. He is a hero and an icon to me, in no small way because of his ability to seamlessly blend being an academic and a yoga practitioner. Because of his authority and for the sake of simplicity, when I needed to look something up while writing this book, I turned to either Feuerstein's *Encyclopedia of Yoga and Tantra* (2011) or *The Yoga*

Tradition: Its History, Literature, Philosophy and Practice. 3rd Ed. (2008).

This book tells the story of how I (mostly) overcame anxiety. The first chapter starts us off at the bottom of my personal barrel. I share this part of my story here because when I was suffering it was helpful to me to read about other people's experiences with anxiety. I didn't feel so alone. Mood disorders are uniquely personal. Maybe you'll be able to identify with some of my experiences, maybe you won't. Maybe reading about someone else's anxiety would trigger anxiety in you. If that's the case, feel free to skip chapter one completely.

Part One: Yoga for Relaxation covers slowing down using progressive relaxation and breathing exercises. In Part Two: Yoga for Self-Acceptance, we encounter a couple of different maps of the psycho-spiritual terrain and move onto the yoga mat. And Part Three: Yoga for Fearlessness goes directly to the source of anxiety—the mind and its thoughts.

I teach people yoga and I teach people how to teach yoga. I write and give workshops on the history, philosophy, and practice of yoga and meditation. I'm not a doctor or a trained healer of any kind. I'm just a friend on the journey. Yoga cannot cure everything and should not replace professional help when that is called for. Yoga is a practice, a way of seeing the world and being in the world that can bring a sense of calm and increase our capacity for compassion toward ourselves and others. My guiding motivation as a teacher is to help people find peace, maybe just for a moment, maybe creating a foundation for something more lasting. That's my wish for this book too, that everyone who reads these words comes away with more peace, more joy, and more love in their lives.

PART ONE

YOGA FOR RELAXATION

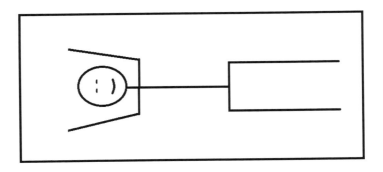

1

HITTING A NEW LOW

My heart is racing. My palms are sweating. I can hardly focus on the cars speeding around me. *Should I or shouldn't I? Should I or shouldn't I?* It's agonizing. *I don't know what to do.* My breath is shallow and fast. Every muscle in my body is tense. Pulling into the parking lot, tears well in my eyes. I can't do it.

I can't do it.

"I'm sorry, sweetie. We can't go to the store," I confess to the child in my backseat. "Mom's having a panic attack."

No French bread with dinner. I berate myself all the way home. *How ridiculous! Afraid of the grocery store. What a loser. I can't believe this,* this *is my life.*

Wearing the Crazy Pants

At 30 I was in a loving marriage, had a bright, beautiful child, and worked at the job I thought I wanted. There was a problem though. The world was closing in on me.

The list of things I couldn't do was growing. I couldn't be around crowds, which at first meant movie theaters on opening day or anything at a stadium. Eventually, it grew to include any movie times, large family gatherings, the grocery store after 10 a.m., and the group of moms watching their kids at gymnastics. I couldn't go anywhere new by myself. I avoided people I didn't know. Then I started avoiding people I *did* know.

When the doorbell rang, I froze like a scared rabbit. I stood in place, my heart pounding, holding my breath until they gave up and went away. I turned down the ringer on my phone so I wouldn't even know when people were calling.

Driving had its own constellation of fears and rituals. I wouldn't drive anywhere I might have felt trapped, so drive-throughs, carwashes, and parking garages were out. I stopped listening to music and sat bolt upright, on high alert. I would check my rearview constantly, certain that I was irritating someone and they were going to confront me. I couldn't drive in heavy traffic, or on a highway, or in the elementary school parking lot, or at night. And as a bonus, I worried obsessively that one of my tires was low. I checked each of them every time I got into or out of the car.

At this point, I taught philosophy at a community college. Always an academic, this should have been a good fit for me. Only it wasn't, because my perfectionism wouldn't let it be. I never measured up to my own expectations. I thought I should know everything about everything I taught, which is impossible in a survey course. I couldn't stand criticism, even coming from students who didn't know jack about philosophy or teaching. I feared missing a mistake while grading papers, so I scrutinized them, spending far more time on each one than was necessary. And, when the monthly bipolar bouts started, work was the first victim.

I know, bipolar doesn't happen within the span of a month. I didn't have bipolar. What I had was a severe anxiety disorder exacerbated by PMS. For two weeks I'd be "fine," full of energy and ideas. I'd sign up for things and start projects. Then for two weeks I'd be depressed. I would cry. No, I would *bawl*. I felt worthless and desperately sad. I would cancel anything I'd signed up for and abandon any projects.

So, that's a start at what I couldn't do—drive, work, be around people. But there's a whole other side of things I *had* to do. I *had* to be *virtuous*. Simplicity, hard work, frugality, strength, charity, intelligence, altruism, environmental awareness—these ideas took over my life.

It would start innocently. I would come up with a question based in reality such as, "How can we live on one income?" Then I would read everything I could find, in this case on simplicity and frugality, and base unbreakable rules on what I learned. I had rules about everything. For instance, I couldn't do laundry when it rained or was windy, because I *had* to use the clothes line. Using the dryer was wasteful and therefore increased my anxiety. Impulse buys were forbidden, as was driving anywhere I could walk, ordering any drink besides water at a restaurant, flushing the toilet more than was absolutely necessary, and using electric gadgets when hand powered ones existed. Reading fiction and watching TV were a waste of time. Every action carried moral significance, and I judged my own and everyone else's actions by these irrational and impossible standards.

Listing my symptoms like this makes them seem pretty abstract. Living them was, well, crazy. Carrying that anxiety in my body made my muscles cramp and my head ache. My face was constantly scrunched up with my brow furrowed and lips either pressed tightly together or pulled all the way into my mouth. I developed TMJ and an underbite! At night I fell asleep exhausted only to wake up a few hours later, my mind whirling. I was *always* on full alert. If other people were in the house, I wasn't just aware of them; it was as if a part of my consciousness was in whichever room they were in.

Imagine working for the grumpiest boss ever: stressed out, sleep deprived, alternately manic and depressed, irritated at even the *idea* of a drop of a hat, and a perfectionist slave driver. That was what it was like inside my brain. I can only apologize for what it was like for the people in my life. I changed my mind, a lot. I threw things. I stopped conversations in the middle and walked away. The silent treatment was my art form. When I did talk about "problems" (which for the most part were delusions of paranoia) I had ruminated, scripted, and rehearsed for hours if not days. I have so much regret that I didn't find help sooner.

I was sore. I was tired. I was scared. I knew I was way out of balance. Somewhere along the way, I had picked up the idea that I should be able to fix myself, that any other course of action would be weak and therefore immoral. I was well and truly trapped. I wish I could say, "And then I found yoga!" at this point. But no, yoga wasn't in my future for a little bit longer. What I can say is I realized I had to make a change. I couldn't live like this, trapped in my house, in fear, in pain.

I needed to change. So I did what I had always done. I read.

Anxiety is the Answer!

I was at the Oregon coast with my extended family when I read the book that would lead to the first chapter in my recovery. *What You Can Change and What You Can't: the Complete Guide to Successful Self-Improvement* is the endearingly clunky title of the book by Martin Seligman that opened my eyes to what was really going on. In the chapter titled "Everyday

Anxiety" there is a brief quiz that asks the reader to score phrases according to how well they describe you. These were statements like "I feel nervous and restless" and "I feel like a failure."

I got a perfect score! I was excited. I had found a clue to what was so very wrong with me. I rushed out to where my sister and father were sitting in the kitchen.

"The coffee tasted like hot dog water," my sister was saying.

"I made that coffee," I said. She looked bewildered. I realize now that she was telling a story. I thought then that she was talking about the coffee they were drinking. I, true to crazy form, could not believe how insensitive she was being and left immediately, without telling anyone of my discovery. I went back to my room and cried.

Being crazy isn't half as fun as the movies make it out to be. I felt raw, exposed, skinless. More *Hellraiser*, less Alex Grey. There were plenty of times when I hoped I'd just die. I didn't want to kill myself and leave my husband and son to deal with that for the rest of their lives. But an accident? That would be all right. Something quick, like a straight on collision. I started envisioning cars coming up on the sidewalk and taking me out when I walked the dog. Or giant trucks running red lights and t-boning my car.

Other times I wished I was a drug addict. Then I wouldn't care about anything except getting high. They could put me in rehab, where someone would feed me and tell me what to do—take all my decisions away. That would be ok. It wasn't until I started feeling a little better that the thought of checking in to a treatment center occurred to me, and by then I was too well.

Beginning Yoga

Everything I read about anxiety said yoga, yoga! Go! Do it! But I had hang ups. First of all, according to my college Hinduism teacher (whose opinion I revered), here were all these know-nothing skinny girls co-opting the sacred tradition of millions of people and turning it into a fitness routine. Way to be part of the American Imperialist machine! (I may be paraphrasing.) Second, if I was going to exercise, I was going to push hard and sweat. Stretching was something you did to cool down, if there was time. What's the point if it's slow?

Only, every single book and article and website said the same thing and I was willing to try anything. I looked up yoga classes in town but I didn't go to any. I was afraid of not knowing what I was doing and of not being able to hear. I had needed hearing aids since I was fourteen but couldn't make myself take the hearing test.

I ordered a yoga DVD and I did that DVD over and over until I had it memorized. I came across a few other videos on Netflix. And eventually I discovered online classes. Yoga became a central aspect of my fitness life. Unfortunately, I treated it like everything else—as a challenge, as something to be eaten whole, without chewing. It was three years from deciding to start yoga to the time when I could get myself to go to a class.

Learning How to Breathe

Along with starting yoga, I quit caffeine, I did an hour of cardio every day, I ate a healthy, plant-based diet, and I tried to meditate—all on the advice of books I'd read about anxiety. And while these things made a dent in my tension (or maybe they just kept me distracted from it), they took all of my energy. I spent all day every day doing maintenance to keep myself from boiling over. And I still boiled over more than I wanted to. I needed help. But how is a person supposed to get help when she's afraid of the phone? I went online, several times, and researched my options for treatment. There were maybe five counselors in our little town who accepted our insurance plan. I researched them all as much as I could and settled on one.

All I had to do was call.

I didn't. I couldn't. I would stare at the phone and tighten up, tears would come, and I would turn my attention elsewhere.

Around this time I found the *Relaxation and Stress Reduction Workbook*. Chapter three is about breathing. What? I know how to breathe; otherwise I'd be dead, right? But I stuck with it because I had to do something and because not finishing a book I had started made me a quitter and was immoral. So, in a way I can thank my own irrational thinking for pushing me toward health.

Eventually, I would realize that what I learned from this book was *pranayama*, the yogic practice of breath control. The first exercise was to lie on the floor in the "dead body" position, *savasana* in yogic terms, and watch my breath. Abdominal breathing, progressive relaxation, and alternate nostril breathing (*nadi shodana*) rounded out the chapter.

Spending even a few minutes laying on the floor breathing was aggravating. I had no patience. But I decided to persevere when I learned that our side ribs are supposed to move when we breathe. Mine didn't. My breathing had been so shallow for so long that my intercostal muscles (the muscles that are supposed to open and close the ribs sort of like a paper lantern) didn't work anymore. That was alarming.

Besides relearning how to breath, progressive relaxation also turned out to be pivotal. I had forgotten what it felt like not to be actively holding myself together at all times. I feared that if I let go physically, I would crumble mentally and just go stark raving insane. Something about relaxing this way, in a circumscribed place and time, made it so I was able to just be, for a minute or two at a time. Then I would spring up and go do some "real work."

After weeks of learning to relax my body and slow down my breath, I was able to make the call. My first choice didn't work out, which crushed me. The next call was a little easier. In fact, it wasn't until the fourth therapist I met that I found a good match for me, which is lucky because I was running out of options. Along the way I was gently yet persistently persuaded to "just try" anti-anxiety medication. I fought the idea but eventually I had suffered enough.

Drugs

I was dead-set against taking medication. I was not going to let Big Pharma turn me into a zombie. I could fix this myself. I'm strong. I'm smart. I'm not *that* sick. I had plenty of reasons, all of them stemming from my irrational need to be "better than that." I've since discovered that this is a common reaction against psychotropics.

In yoga, as we will see, the body is considered a vehicle and the mind is part of the body. If your leg was broken, you would get a cast. If your skin broke out in sores, you would use a salve and take antibiotics. Physical diseases and disorders are rarely seen as the product of a lack of willpower. But for some reason we think we should be able to take care of mental disorders on our own. Minds can be broken, disordered, diseased. I would never advocate drugs to anyone who didn't need them. But I absolutely recommend them for people who are suffering. I would either be a raging alcoholic or dead without them. (Fluvoxamine works well for me. It wasn't the first I tried. Like many, I had to experiment with a few types to find the one that fits my brain best.)

The first couple days on anti-anxiety drugs were

whacky. I was tired and spacey—stoned, really. Some people refer to this as the zombie phase. But for me, the relief was awesome. It had been ages since I'd felt anything approaching *Aw, who gives a shit?* or *Meh, it'll take care of itself.* I felt a childlike glee at hearing those types of thoughts again. I completely stopped all exercise except yoga, because, you know, whatever.

The honeymoon didn't last, though. Meds don't change your personality, just your chemistry. After about a week, my brain adjusted to the new levels. I plateaued somewhere south of completely stressed. From this new vantage point I was able to observe my own thoughts without getting caught up in them. Talk about disturbing! And, while it was scary to realize how irrational my thoughts had become, I knew I was on the right path.

With the help of medication, therapy, and my home yoga practice, I made a list of things I feared doing and started doing them. I got hearing aids and I went to my first yoga class (with my sister). The following chapters tell the rest of the story, how yoga has helped me gain control of my emotions, change my thought patterns, and create new habits.

Yoga is an ever expanding phenomenon, spread over thousands of years, various fields of human inquiry, and now every continent. What I present here is admittedly piecemeal. I hope that for those who are already interested in yoga, these pages will deepen your understanding and open new doors. And for those who are just getting started, whom I address throughout, this will serve as a meaningful introduction, which not only provides practical solutions to your problems with anxiety but also sparks an interest in learning more about the boundless, fascinating, kaleidoscopic wonder that is yoga.

2

FEAR

Anxiety comes from fear. Humans evolved the ability to fear for the same reason every other self-respecting mammal did: survival. We fear things that will hurt us. However, since we are social creatures we don't just fear physical injury. We fear that we will miss something important, look stupid, lose something we love, or have to do something we hate, among countless other things. Even though these fears are very different than the fear we experience in a dangerous situation, our bodies only have the one central nervous system with which to respond.

Usually fear of physical injury is short lived. Oh-dear-God-that-truck's-coming-right-at-whew-that-was-close! Adrenalin and cortisol are released, heart rate rises, extremities may tingle as the blood vessels open to accommodate the rush of blood, eyes get wide, breath becomes shallow; we go through the whole sympathetic nervous system dance. And then it resolves. It may take a few minutes to shake the rush as the parasympathetic system restores equilibrium, but it passes.

These other fears—of failure, of shame, of loss—don't come at us like a speeding truck and they don't resolve themselves like a "near miss" either. They build slowly and they linger. Each time we have an anxiety-producing thought we get a little dose of adrenalin, a little hit of cortisol. Here's the hook, they're energizing. They're supposed to be, to give us the energy to escape a tiger or to wrestle our baby away from a bear. In little doses, we don't feel that escalation, that peak and resolution. We just get a little high.

You can see where this is going. Anxiety, as uncomfortable as it may be, can be addictive. If a person has been living with elevated levels of adrenalin and cortisol for weeks or months or years, they've built up a tolerance. Their stress level becomes their maintenance dose. We all have people in our lives who really light up at the first sign of trouble, if not tragedy. They are in their element when things are going wrong. I can't speak for every case, but maybe some of these folks are just getting a chemical jolt from the chaos.

Like most drug addictions, stress and anxiety have side effects: weight gain or loss, insomnia, muscle tightness, irritability, distractibility, memory failure, frequent urge to pee, high blood pressure, and so on. And like most drug addictions, the cure is not to treat the symptoms but the source: fear.

Skeletons

For most of my life I felt wrong, out of place, lost. In high school, my punk rock salad days, I became interested in counter cultures and the history of going against the grain. The Transcendentalists, bohemians, and beatniks were my favorite topics of study. It wasn't a stretch from there to Eastern mysticism.

At 19, absolutely smitten with the Buddhist take on fearlessness, I found a meditation in Tarthan Tulku's *Openness Mind*. In this practice, the goal is to visualize yourself as a skeleton. After death and decay, all that is left is the bones. Sitting with my bones day after day, at a very impressionable age, did indeed engender fearlessness and also detachment.

Detachment and compassion are the two attitudes toward life the yogic worldview encourages us to adopt. Detachment means simply stepping back and observing, becoming a witness to the world and one's own mind. Detachment needs to be balanced with compassion, otherwise we risk becoming unfeeling automatons.

At 19 I lacked the balance that came from compassion. Fearlessness became recklessness. Dispassion became cold-heartedness. I disengaged from the world. It felt safe but unfulfilling. I still think the skeleton meditation is a great exercise. It's a meaningful practice to remember the sticks and stones that hold us upright. At 19, I just was not ready.

I mention this episode here as we transition into the causes of suffering because these two dispositions, detachment and compassion, weave their way through everything else we will talk about.

Klesha

According to Patanjali's *Yoga Sutras*, there are five *klesha* or causes of affliction. *Klesha* translates from Sanskrit as "poison." According to yoga, all human suffering can be attributed to one of these five *klesha*: lack of knowledge, confusion about the ego, attachment, aversion, and the will to live. I'll explain.

The first *klesha* or cause of suffering is *avidya*. *Vidya* means spiritual knowledge and the "a-" in front of it signifies "lack of." *Avidya* is often translated as *ignorance*, but with "ignore" right in there, I think ignorance ascribes too much willfulness. Really, we are misinformed, maybe even mislead, and therefore mistaken. The knowledge we lack is how to distinguish between what is Real and Eternal and what is changing and therefore temporary. In yogic terms, what is Real and Eternal is called Brahman, what we might call the Sacred, Spirit, the Divine, or God, and this is the Eternal Conscious Awareness that permeates the universe and everything in it.

Problems (afflictions, suffering) arise when we mistake the temporary for the Eternal and give things that are transitory the importance of the Sacred.

Remember those *Don't Sweat the Small Stuff . . . and It's All Small Stuff* books? It's like that. At some level we know that everything is always in a very real way on its way out. Days pass, things wear out and fall apart, children become grownups, and everybody eventually dies. This life is temporary, as is everything in it. We are trying to tap into this understanding when we ask "How much will this matter in five years?"

With *vidya*, or spiritual knowledge, we are able to keep perspective. *Avidya* is said to be the root cause of all forms of suffering.

The second *klesha* is *asmita*, which translates into the awkward expression "I-am-ness." What is struggling to be described here is the perception of *being* the ego, the "I." It's easy enough to fall into this misperception just through how we experience the world, but in our market- and marketing-driven culture, it can be hard to see past.

Here's the key—you *have* an ego. You are not your ego.

Egos, or senses of self, change. They change with time, with growth, with trauma, with hard knocks to the head. The sense of self is a conglomeration of personality traits, memories, likes and dislikes, and they are part of the vehicle—a by-product of inhabiting a human body with a functioning brain. But, with *vidya*, we recognize that the sense of self is not solid or forever and the ego softens its death-grip on us.

Brahman (or the Sacred) is sometimes translated as

the Self, with a capital S. It is often said that the goal of the spiritual journey is discovering the Self within. The trick is distinguishing the self with a lowercase "s" from the Self with a capital "S."

Important! We are not trying to get rid of the ego. Everybody needs an ego. Egos make decisions and keep us safe. At 19, when I tried to bypass building a strong ego and go straight to detachment, I got lost. My sense of self was not strong enough to gracefully retreat. Instead of building a connection to my Self, my ego morphed into someone "above it all" and beyond the trivialities of the everyday. In other words, a cold-hearted jerk.

A weak ego will fight tooth and nail for center stage. A strong ego can step aside, gracefully allowing Spirit to unfold.

Raga means attachments and is the third *klesha*. This is the category of things we love, things we like, and things of which we are fond. Here we find the events we would prefer to see happen, the people we would like to always have in our lives, and the objects we own or want to own. But whatever they are, they never do last. And when something doesn't work out, when things break or people go away, we suffer loss, disappointment, envy, and so on.

What we misunderstand when we try to make these attachments permanent, the center of our lives, is that they are by nature impermanent. They are just as transitory as spring flowers and sand paintings. It is not that we shouldn't appreciate and be grateful for the good things in life but that it is misguided to cling to them. The aim is to let them come and let them go.

The goal is similar with the next *klesha*, *dvesha*. This is the category of aversions. It covers all the things we hate, things that are annoying, embarrassing, shameful, guilt-inducing—everything we wish was otherwise. And the advice is the same as for attachments: let them come and let them go. Trying to avoid those situations that make us anxious only serves to reinforce the aversion.

Attachments and aversions are based in fear: they are the things we fear happening, fear losing, fear having to face, fear having to do without. The final *klesha*, *abhiniveshah* taps what for many is the ultimate fear, the fear of death. *Abhiniveshah* means the will to stay alive. This is a special case of attachment (to life) and aversion (to death). Patanjali, the author of this list of *klesha*, assures us that the will to live is present "even in the wise." Without compassion, detaching from the will to live would look the same as giving up. Accepting the reality of death with detached compassion is very different than being resigned to fate.

There are positive and negative ways to detach from attachments and aversions, and the difference between them is compassion. It may be possible to let go of likes and dislikes by simply cutting off. Some of us experience this quite involuntarily, when the world is just too overwhelming and the best defense is to just shut down. But that isn't what we are trying to get at here. Detachment, balanced by compassion, is a matter of perspective. It is the recognition that "this too shall pass." And that we are all in the same boat, not just other people but ourselves too; each of us experiences the highs and lows of life. Detached compassion requires accepting our humanness, our limitations and frailty. Everyone, as they say, has their story. It very well may be that it is only when we can find that paradoxical balance of dispassionate compassion that unconditional love is possible. The first paradox of many!

To briefly recap, in the yogic view life is filled with suffering because we misunderstand the Spiritual Reality of which we are a part. Failing to recognize the difference between the Eternal and the temporary, we develop aversions and attachments to people, things, events, etc. Because of these preferences, we move through life like the ball in a pinball game, getting batted around, banging into things, and occasionally falling into a dark hole and having to start over. The solution to this problem is to develop detachment and compassion. And this, at long last, is the antidote to fear: we have to be willing to let the vicissitudes of life come and go with an open heart and an accepting attitude.

Yeah, that's great. And just how do we get from shopping for crazy pants to that kind of equanimity? The adventure begins by slowing down.

3

SLOWING DOWN

Throughout the history of yoga, there have been analogies made between driving a horse and carriage and being a human. The carriage itself is said to represent the body. The horse, which is wild and unwieldy, is the mind. And the driver is the higher Self, who must first yoke (which comes from the same root word, *yuj*, as yoga) the horse and then train it.

To modernize this analogy and make it relevant to our topic, anxiety can feel a lot like being at the wheel of a runaway car: no brakes, no steering, veering whichever way the bumps in the road dictate, and going fast! Here, instead of the horse, the engine is the mind, and the first thing to do is slow it down.

Why is slowing down so difficult? Everyone has to find their own answer to this. Maybe it's cultural. According to the marketplace, faster is better. From phones to fast food, we expect speed. The desire to succeed, *to get ahead*, is planted deep when we are young, and achievement and success are defined in objective terms like how much more you have than others. Here's something: as an autonomous grownup, you get to define achievement and success however you want! Speed is not mandatory. Some people thrive on it but for many of us, we just feel hurried and harried and worn down.

Maybe we're afraid to slow down because we've simply grown into what we thought people expected. Especially women are told they will have to take on many roles (worker, partner, mother, etc.) and will have to multitask. If perfectionism is part of your experience, then each of these roles fights for dominance as you move through the day. Here's another thing: multitasking is a sham. It's less efficient, less productive, and more stressful. Whenever you can, do one thing at a time and give that activity your full attention.

Some people can't stand to slow down because that's when the judgmental thoughts come to the surface.

Whatever the reason we sped up in the first place, it's where we are now. Even at my most reclusive, I still felt I had to be busy. It showed I was important, contributing; I wasn't a slacker. Doing nothing was morally reprehensible. Anytime I was still, I started to fidget and eventually panic. Long lines, waiting in the car, being ready to leave too early—all were skinpickingly aggravating. (Picking was my compulsive release valve.)

There are lots of ways to slow down. A walk in the sunshine, getting down on the floor with the dog or cat, or getting a massage from someone you love are nice ways to take a break. But we are looking for something more lasting and something that comes from the inside out. The following practices tackle this first and foremost issue of slowing down.

Practice *Relaxing*

Anxiety thrives in the feedback loop between the body and the mind. A signal from the mind tenses the body and tension from the body signals the mind that there is something to fear. This first practice, a type of progressive relaxation, begins to disable that loop. Relaxing the body eases the production of stress-related hormones and neurotransmitters.

Is progressive relaxation yoga? Well, in the 1920s Edmund Jacobson M.D. developed something he called Progressive Muscle Relaxation. And also in the twenties Paramhansa Yogananda brought the Yogoda system of exercise from India, the first step of which is to relax by gently tightening and releasing each body part. There was a considerable amount of cross-fertilization between cultures when it came to exercise and "physical culture" in the early decades of the 1900s. Whether the Indians gave it to the Americans or vice versa, it is part of yoga now and it's extraordinarily effective.

The benefits of progressive relaxation are many. Right away you will feel a sense of relief from tension. Your heart and breathing rates will ease. More than that, in progressive relaxation the body becomes the object of meditation. For those of us with anxiety, sitting to meditate can seem torturous. Every moment of "stillness" is another chance to listen to the inner diatribe of what we aren't getting done, what we need to fix, what terrible thing is just around the corner, what we need to do as soon as this is over, *dear God, is it over yet? Please, please let it be over already.* With each of those thoughts, anxiety builds, tension builds, and we can end up worse off than when we began. But in this technique, the mind is occupied. It doesn't get the chance to unravel.

The first step for many of us in the practice of yoga is relearning how to inhabit the body. That may sound weird but stay with me. Anxiety makes us feel like we live in our heads, always thinking, planning, scripting, worrying, and so on. In progressive relaxation we learn how to shift our awareness from the head and let it move freely about the body. We become reacquainted with our bodies, maybe even learning something new.

Simply put, in progressive relaxation we direct our attention toward various parts of the body, lingering for a few breaths at each location while sending that body part the suggestion to relax. I will lead you through this in more detail soon. There are several different techniques for this exercise. If you would prefer a more guided experience, try searching the Internet with the keywords "progressive relaxation audio." You are guaranteed to find several free options.

There are two basic levels of progressive relaxation. In the first, each muscle group is tightened and then released with the intention of complete relaxation. In the second, we forego tightening the muscles and move straight to relaxing. I would recommend trying them both at least once. Then you can know which one works best for you.

It may seem counterintuitive to try to further tighten your muscles if you are already really tense. There is a point to it. It shows the body the difference between tighter and looser. Eventually, as far-fetched as this seems, you will find that you can tighten the whole body all at once, release, and truly be relaxed. It's not magic. It's behaviorism. We are pairing the stimulus of tightening with the response of relaxing. It may not be magic but it is *magical*.

Relaxation Practice 1

Progressive relaxation can be done seated or lying down. Either way, make sure you are fully supported. Have a timer nearby. (If you don't like being alerted by the harsh tones of most timers, there are free meditation applications available for smart phones that have gentle chimes.) Allow at least fifteen minutes for this practice, and read through the instructions before you begin.

Warning over-achievers! "Tighten" does not mean squeeze to within an inch of dear life. We are looking for the amount of effort equal to opening a pickle jar, not bending steel bars. Also, if you develop a cramp, release the hold and take that body part through its range of motion until the cramp subsides.

~ Set the timer to one minute. Without starting it, set it aside. (As you become more comfortable in the last steps of this process, you can increase the time to three minutes and then to five.)

~ Settle into your position. Take three deep breaths.

~ Begin with your **toes**. Curl them tightly and count to three at a moderate speed. It's tempting to rush this but that won't help. One Mississippi, two Mississippi, three Mississippi, or something like that. Then release the tension and relax your toes. Take two slow breaths keeping with the intention to relax your toes.

~ Next, pick up your feet and flex your **ankles**, bringing your toes back toward your knees. Feel your feet and calves tighten. Count slowly to three. Then release the tension and relax your feet and calves. Keeping your attention in your feet and lower legs, take two full breaths.

~ Now, engage your **thighs** and glutes (butt muscles). One Mississippi, two Mississippi, three Mississippi. Release, relax. Breathe.

~ Pull in your **stomach** muscles. One . . . two . . . three. Release, relax. Breathe.

~ Hunch your **shoulders** up by your ears. Count to three. Release, relax. Breathe.

~ Make fists with your hands and tighten your hands and **arms**. One . . . two . . . three. Release the tension; relax your hands and arms. Take two full breaths.

~ Shift your awareness to your **face**. Shut your eyes tightly, press your lips together, and scrunch all your facial muscles in toward your nose. Count to three. Release, relax, and take two full breaths.

~ Now, return your awareness to your toes and, working upward, relax any part of your body that may have become tense again.

~ Start the timer. Close your eyes and do what you can to remain physically relaxed and aware of your breath.

~ When the timer sounds, gently blink your eyes open. Take a deep, full, slow breath, and ease back into your day.

You may find that tightening one part of your body leads to tightness in other parts. That's all right. The ability to isolate muscles will come with repetition. Speaking of which, at first, it's best to do this exercise once a day.

Relaxation Practice 2

Did you read right through without stopping to try Relaxation Practice 1? Yep. I knew it, because I'm that annoying guy in the movies who says with all the earnestness he can muster, "Kid, I used to be you." I will get on with Practice 2, but first this: you have to do the work. If you don't change what you are doing, nothing will change. It sounds tautological put that way, but in my own journey I read and read, hoping for that one great A-ha! moment when everything would fall into place and I would spontaneously be well. It doesn't happen. There is work to be done and it is hard work. But it is worthwhile and rewarding, too.

It's cool if you want to read through the chapter or even the whole book before trying any of the practices. It's all right to pick and choose the ones that look like they will work best for you and leave the rest. Yoga has a long tradition of meeting people where they are. There is no dogmatism, no have-tos or or-elses in yoga. Take what works for you.

Onward! If Relaxation Practice 1 didn't work for you, either because it created cramps or just felt wrong to *add* tension to your body, here is another option, which can also be a second step after mastering Practice 1. For this variation of progressive relaxation, again all you need is a comfortable place to be and a timer. This method is a little more mentally demanding. If you find that your thoughts stray from the task at hand, don't worry about it. That's completely normal. Just take that opportunity to practice letting go of those thoughts and return to the last location on which you were focusing.

~ Set your timer to one, three, or five minutes, depending how experienced you are with this exercise. Without starting it, set the timer aside.

~ Get comfortable. Settle in and take three deep, slow breaths.

~ Bring your awareness to your **feet**. Send them the suggestion to relax. Some people find it helpful to imagine knotted rope untying, butter melting, or something that means relax, unwind, and release to you. Take two full, slow breaths while allowing your feet to relax.

~ Next, let your attention settle in your **lower legs**. Invite them to relax. Imagine the muscles growing soft. Take two complete breaths while the lower legs release and relax.

~ Move to your **thighs** and do the same. Let your breath be slow and easy.

~ Then your **hips**, glutes, and pelvis. Even if you don't feel any release this time, you are planting the idea in your hips that one day soon, it would be ok for them to relax.

~ Move to your **back**. Imagine the big and small muscles of your back relaxing outward from your spine. Start with your lower back. Breathe. Then your mid-back. Breathe. And your upper back. Breathe.

~ Now, allow your awareness to settle in your low **belly**. Relax and breathe. Then your **solar plexus** (between the belly button and lower ribs). And then your **chest**. Let your muscles be soft and move with your breath.

~ Bring your attention into your **arms** and hands. Give them the suggestion to relax. Imagine and feel the muscles releasing and softening. Move through two complete breaths.

~ Now your **shoulders**. We hold a lot of stress in our shoulders. They think they are protecting us. Be gentle. Baby steps are still steps. Allow your shoulders to release as much as they can today. Breathe here.

~ Let your **neck** relax.

~ Soften your **face**. The jaw, the muscles around the mouth and eyes, and the forehead are all great places to settle your awareness while you take two breaths.

~ Allow your entire **head** to relax, letting your attention settle around your hairline and around your ears.

~ When your attention has travelled all the way up your body, return to your toes and, working upward, relax any part of your body that may have become tense.

~ Start the timer. Close your eyes and do what you can to remain physically relaxed and aware of your breath.

~ When the timer sounds, blink your eyes open. Take a deep, full, slow breath and ease back into your day.

Practice *Breathing*

Progressive relaxation is an important first step in disabling the anxiety feedback loop between the body and the mind. Conscious breathing, as you've seen, plays a central role. The breath can be seen as the current carrying the feedback signal from the mind to the body and back again. When we feel anxious or threatened, our breath becomes rapid and moves high in the chest. Hopefully, during progressive relaxation, you will find your breath begin to slow and deepen.

Pranayama is the yogic term for breathing exercises. *Prana* means life force, like chi in Chinese medicine and acupuncture. Yogis believe the breath and life force are coterminous but not identical. It's easy to see how they might have come up with this. Life outside the womb begins with an inhale and ends with an exhale. In fact, some yogis believe that between this first inhale and last exhale, each person has a predetermined number of breaths. So the slower we breathe, the longer we live. This makes perfect sense in our time, when stress is involved in so many cases of premature aging and death.

Ayama, the second part of *pranayama*, means "to extend." *Pranayama* is the practice of extending your life by extending your breath. While there are *pranayama* techniques that speed the breath and energize the nervous system, the original yogis were seeking to still the mind by stilling the breath. And while these faster methods have value in other settings, I would not recommend forceful breathing techniques to anyone experiencing anxiety.

Relaxing the body is a prerequisite to *pranayama*, but these exercises don't have to be done lying down. Once they become familiar, the two techniques I'll introduce here can be done standing, which makes them far more useful in public places than progressive relaxation.

Pranayama 1: Abdominal Breathing

Have you ever watched a baby or a cat or dog sleeping? Most likely, you could see them belly breathing. That's how we naturally breathe when we're relaxed. What's happening is that the diaphragm (that's the large, flat, oval muscle that attaches to the bottom of the rib cage) moves down into the stomach region, creating a partial vacuum in the lungs and provoking the inhale. The incoming air fills the lungs which gently compress the organs of the abdomen toward the pelvis, causing the belly to expand. On the exhale, the diaphragm moves up into the lower thoracic cavity, the area between the lower ribs, pressing the air out and allowing the belly to contract.

Abdominal breathing isn't just for babies and puppies. It can be learned (or re-learned), and the main reason to do so is that belly breathing sends the message to the central nervous system that everything is ok. Just as anxiety can make us breathe high in the chest and breathing high in the chest can make us feel anxiety, breathing low in the belly can make us feel calm. This is a great way to interrupt the feedback loop.

Besides anxiety, another reason many of us breathe high in the chest is that we were taught to hold in our stomach. In an effort to look thinner, we have been aggravating our breathing pattern and therefore our anxiety by keeping our stomach muscles contracted.

Relaxing the stomach is the first of many suggestions in this guide that may provoke a struggle between what society teaches and a healthier way of being. Believe me, holding your belly in for vanity's sake isn't worth never overcoming your anxiety.

If it has been a long time since you felt your stomach move with your breath, begin this exercise lying on your back. If this causes discomfort in your lower back, slide a pillow or rolled up blanket under your knees. If it's uncomfortable in your neck and/or jaw, prop your head up on a folded blanket. The higher your head, the more likely your trachea will be partially obstructed, so no fluffy pillows here.

At first, set the timer for three minutes. Later, you can progress to five and then ten minute intervals. During this exercise and the next, stray thoughts will occur. That's normal. That's what brains do; it's their job. Practice letting go of these thoughts. While it's easier said than done, the goal is to notice when you have a thought and decide not to follow it. Return your awareness to the breathing exercise as many times as it takes until the timer sounds. At first this may seem radical and even dangerous. We like to think our thoughts keep us safe. You will be fine. And it's important that you do it. It is the first step toward moving into observational or witness consciousness. If the thought is important, it will come back later.

If you experience a tenacious thought and, after trying to let it go and return your awareness to the breath several times, you find tension is building instead of releasing, stop the timer. Get up, write down the thought, and then continue on with the exercise.

Please remember, if you experience any physical discomfort during these practices, do whatever you need to do to make yourself comfortable. You can even set the technique aside for a few breaths and begin again. Also, while most people find these types of exercises calming, if you experience troublesome mental discomfort, set the technique aside. Not every technique will help every person, but hopefully every person can be helped by some of these techniques. You won't know until you try!

~ Set the timer for three to five minutes and put it aside.

~ Lay comfortably on your back or sit upright. Either way, keep your spine long.

~ Relax. Scan your body for places you feel tightness and use a few breaths to release any tension.

~ Place your dominant hand over your navel and your other hand over the middle of your chest (the heart center). If your elbows are floating, either slide your hands away from center until your elbows and upper arms are supported or use folded blankets to support your upper arms and elbows.

~ Notice where your breath moves your body without doing anything to change it.

~ Allow your breath to become smooth and easy.

~ Shift the movement of your breath into your abdomen. Feel with your hand as your abdomen rises and falls.

~ Your chest may become relatively still. If not, that's ok. It can take practice and time to alter deeply ingrained physical patterns.

~ When your breath is moving your abdomen, start the timer.

~ For the duration of the exercise, take slow, easy breaths that make your belly rise and fall. Notice when thoughts arise. Approach these thoughts with detachment and compassion. Gently release them and return your awareness to the breath.

~ When the timer sounds, stay relaxed and complete the round of breath you are moving through.

~ Then release your breath to its natural rhythm.

~ Notice any differences in the quality of your breath from when you began to this point.

~ After a few slow, calm breaths, gently begin to move your body in whatever way feels best.

~ Ease back into your day.

Pranayama 2: Four-part Breath

Sometimes called square breathing, this *pranayama* introduces the idea of pauses in the breathing cycle. I used to think breathing had two parts, the inhale and the exhale. Turns out, that's just half of it. When we take slow, full, conscious breaths, there is a pause after the inhale and one after the exhale, too.

These pauses may be absent because our breathing is normally so shallow that the body is always asking for "More fresh air, please!" When our breathing is comfortably deep, there is a space where the circulatory system is sated, when, for just a brief moment, we don't need to be pulling new air in or pushing old air out. We can use that space to begin to experience stillness, maybe even peace.

Physically, this technique helps slow down the nervous system. Mentally, it increases our ability to concentrate. It can be done lying down or seated. I would suggest lying down if you are still learning progressive relaxation and abdominal breathing.

~ Set the timer for three to five minutes and put it aside.

~ Find a comfortable position, seated or lying down. Either way, keep the spine long rather than rounded.

~ Scan your body for anywhere there might be tension. Use a few breaths to relax.

~ Settle your awareness on your breath. Just witness its movements for at least three breaths.

~ Allow your breath to become slow and easy.

~ Notice the short pauses at the top of the inhale and at the bottom of the exhale. Elongate those pauses by a second or two.

~ Start the timer.

At this point, you are doing the four-part breath. In the beginning, let this be your practice for at least a few days. After that, see if you like the following additions, which turn this into square breathing.

~ Begin counting 1-2 during each stage of the breathing cycle. Inhale 1-2, pause 1-2, exhale 1-2, pause 1-2, and repeat.

~ Eventually work your way up to a count of 1-2-3-4 during each stage.

~ When the timer sounds, stay with the round (or square) of breath you are moving through. Then release any effort to control your breath.

~ Notice any differences between your breath now and when you began.
~ After a few slow breaths, begin to move your body. Stretch out.
~ Ease back into your day.

What's Next?

In this chapter we have talked about how to slow down the run away car that is anxiety. In the next chapter, we will pull over and pop the hood. We'll also dig through the glove compartment to find some maps of the territory.

PART TWO

YOGA FOR
SELF-ACCEPTANCE

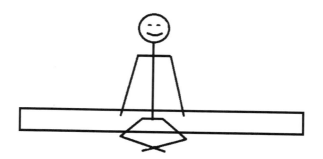

4

MAPS

While I don't advertise them as such, every yoga class I teach is for stress-relief and self-acceptance. Often, when I make this overtly clear, someone will stay after class and share their story. This week, it happened three times! I truly appreciate when people feel safe enough to share with me. It makes me feel like I'm in the right place, doing the right work.

Talking about anxiety and mood disorders in general is tough. Especially when we are in the throes of one, we fear being stigmatized. I assure you, this is no reason not to talk about it. First of all, most people are not really jerks. Secondly, millions of us have stress, anxiety, or depression. Over one in four adults in the U.S. has experienced a mood disorder. Those are pretty good empathy odds.

For the most part, what you think people are thinking is an assumption based on your own fear and self-criticism. There may in fact be some haters in your life, people who do actually tell you "It's all your head" and that you should "Pull yourself up by your bootstraps," whatever those are. In either case, imagined or real, I find it helpful to turn to the sage words of modern day spiritual pioneer RuPaul Charles: "What other people think of me is none of my damn business!" Let's say it again, "What other people think of me is none of my damn business!"

And that, dear reader, is liberating!

Urban Apes

When we evolved on the savannah, we adapted to small bands of 30 to 50 people. While we can't know for certain, research on present-day hunter-gatherer tribes suggests early humans probably worked an average of five hours a day and spent the rest of their time socializing and getting stoned in hammocks. (I'm not a hundred percent on that last part.) Our needs were simple: food, shelter, and safety from predators.

Life was short, in no small part because as animals go we are ridiculous with our big heads and soft skin. By standing upright, we might as well wear our internal organs on the outside. So eventually, humans started joining together into bigger groups, trading uncertainty and fear for safety and, for many, subjugation.

The point is we did not evolve to live surrounded by strangers, with our eyes and ears constantly bombarded by images and language, or to move at 80 miles an hour, either literally or metaphorically. It's baffling to me that we aren't all completely bananas!

So, while the haters will hate for whatever reasons they come up with, anxiety is a perfectly normal reaction to the situation into which we were born. That said, it's not an excuse to stay anxious. What we do have as members of this species are big brains and along with that can come smarts. As individuals, we can use our smarts to alter our environments, retrain our nervous systems, and restructure our brains to manage the sensory overload we face every day.

The Seven Stages of Psycho-Spiritual Growth

On a journey, few things are quite as useful as a map. The seven stages of psycho-spiritual growth is a map that helped guide me out of some very dark territory. Just as in the discussion of the *klesha* (causes of suffering), this is an overview, a bird's eye view of the terrain. Right now, it may feel like you need all of your effort just to put one foot in front of the other. I offer this list not to push or hurry you. Everybody's process is unique and, while no one can tell you how long any stage of healing ought to take, I firmly believe that slow progress with steady commitment wins the day. I offer what follows as a beacon, a light in the distance to help set the course.

Georg Feuerstein, who was perhaps the preeminent yogic scholar of our time, developed the seven stages of psycho-spiritual growth based on a lifetime of study.

What follows is centered on his description of the stages in the audio book *The Lost Teachings of Yoga* (2003). All of the quotations below are from Feuerstein and were transcribed by me. (When you're reading them, try to imagine them carefully enunciated with a German accent.) The stages are as follows: self-observation, self-acceptance, self-understanding, self-discipline, self-actualization, self-transcendence, and self-transformation. I'll discuss each briefly here and in more depth throughout the rest of the book.

Stage One: Self-observation

In this stage we begin to ask ourselves, *Why am I doing what I am doing? What am I thinking? How am I feeling?* "The emphasis in self-observation," says Feuerstein, "is on being consciously present." This is the budding of mindfulness.

To begin, we must exchange the discomfort of living with a barrage of negative automatic thoughts that may be just on the periphery of consciousness for the discomfort of becoming completely aware of them. This will start to happen of its own accord as you begin to slow down. At this stage a journal in which to write down your insights is a valuable tool. Just putting your thoughts on paper can help you gain perspective.

Stage Two: Self-acceptance

As we start to pay attention to our habits of thought and action, what we find can be alarming. Regardless of how irrational or disheartening or even infuriating our discoveries, the work of this stage is to accept ourselves exactly as we are, right now. This is easier when we remember that the body and mind are "not who we are in essence." You are not your thoughts. You are something much greater. Thoughts are temporary. Compassion and detachment are crucial to cultivate at this stage. Feuerstein says, "We should look at our negative emotions and patterns as objectively and dispassionately as we look at a freckle on the body. In other words, we identify with them as little as we would identify with a freckle."

Self-acceptance shouldn't be confused with doing nothing. "Our present condition is the direct outcome of our past mental activity. We can't change the past. We can only change the future. And we can change the future by acting differently right now, in the present."

Stage Three: Self-understanding

At this stage we come to perceive the significance of what we've discovered in the first two stages. In Feuerstein's words, "It's necessary for us to know not only how but why we act and react in predictable ways." To this end, community is vital. Many of us may need a trained listener in the form of a counselor or therapist. Some just need someone empathic enough to act as a sounding board and provide perspective. Being part of a community of fellow travelers also helps provide that perspective.

How will we know when we're making progress? "I think we are maturing in the stage of self-understanding," says Feuerstein, "when we can freely acknowledge that we are somewhat ridiculous creatures, when we can start laughing about ourselves. I believe humor and self-understanding go hand in hand."

Stage Four: Self-discipline

Habits are tenacious. It takes hard work and dedication to replace them. According to Feuerstein, that's exactly what self-discipline is: "Self-discipline is conscious repetition of desirable forms of behavior as opposed to the unconscious repetition that marks our conventional life."

It is easy to get bogged down or possibly even bored with this stage. It takes discipline to stick with the practices that will make the changes first easier and then permanent. "Self-discipline," he assures us, "sets up counter habits, more benign grooves, that slowly move us in the direction of enlightenment, inner freedom."

We continue to practice: to come to the mat, to sit in stillness, to observe, accept, and understand with detachment and compassion. The rewards do come. "Regular yogic discipline makes us glow like the sun, and then we can offer warmth and life to our fellow beings."

Stage Five: Self-actualization

Self-discipline leads to discovering our untapped potential. We begin to blossom, eventually growing into the best version of our potential selves.

This stage often gets short shrift in yoga, if not overlooked completely. This is due in part to the misunderstanding that we are trying to overcome and subdue the ego. In reality, we need strong egos. That is to say, we need to have a sense of competency, faith in our abilities to successfully contend with anything life puts in our path. As I mentioned before, a weak ego will claw and fight to stay in the limelight. Only a fully developed ego can graciously cede the attention of center stage.

Stage Six: Self-transcendence

Self-transcendence is less a stage than an experience. "Yoga is interested in us," Feuerstein explains, "as infinite, super-conscious, immortal Spirit. It wants to take us out of our conventional grooves into no grooves at all." Self-transcendence then is the ecstatic state of *samadhi*, of Union.

Ecstatic self-transcendence is the outcome of commitment to practice. Of the many forms *samadhi* can take, the highest is the state of formless ecstasy, *nirvikalpa samadhi*. "*Nirvikalpa samadhi*, this higher form of *samadhi*, is the narrow gate through which we can enter into full enlightenment, our true nature." We will talk more about *samadhi* in chapter eight.

Stage Seven: Self-transformation

This is living enlightenment. An exceedingly rare occurrence, the person who reaches this state is One with everything. It is said that when a person is completely enlightened, they are able to manifest what we would consider paranormal powers with ease. And at this highest of all levels, the adept can transubstantiate the material body into light.

Back to earth! It's tempting to approach any list like this with pen in hand, ready to tick the box and move on to the next stage. But the journey of self-development lasts a lifetime and the stages are not discreet. While observation has to happen before acceptance and actualization before transformation, the path continuously loops back on itself.

Observation, aka mindfulness, is the ground of which the path is made, the yellow bricks of the yellow brick road. Usually, mindfulness is quickly followed by the word "meditation." And we will get there. However, in my experience, anxiety can make meditation excruciating. When your thoughts are rapid-fire, irrational, and self-defeating, sitting still can be brutal. Since we aren't in the business of making things worse, we need to find a different place to practice observation. The physical practice of yoga is a powerful tool when it comes to building mindfulness.

Pulling Over

As the first step on the path, self-observation deserves special attention. To return to the metaphor of the mind as a runaway car, when we begin in earnest to figure out what's causing our anxiety, once we've slowed down, we really should pull over and pop the hood. Few of us can actually take a break from all of our responsibilities, all at once. It's important, though, to do what you can to step off the race track for a while. Take as long as you need, at least a week, without making any changes or taking on new obligations. Show extraordinary compassion toward yourself and don't do anything you don't want to do, as long as your actions don't put yourself or others in harm's way.

The first time I "pulled over," it felt wrong. I thought I was being selfish and that people would judge me as lazy. Try to resist the urge to keep in the swing of things. It may sound trite but you have to take care of yourself first, and no one else is going to do it for you. If you want to feel joy and peace again, if you want to be a better friend, lover, parent, whatever you want to be good at, if you want a shot at a long and healthy life, take this time now.

Samskara and Karma

Now to look under the hood. During this time, pause often to ask yourself, *What am I doing? Why am I doing it? What am I thinking? What am I feeling?* Many of our motivations are unconscious. These deep habits of thought are things we've learned along the way, behaviors that have been reinforced one way or another even though they don't serve our best interests. In yogic lingo, these habits are called *samskara*, imprints in the subconscious created by experience. As long as we are motivated by *samskara*, we continue to create *karma*.

Translated literally, *karma* means "action." The way we're referring to it here, it is the principle of causality. Our thoughts and actions have repercussions on a sort of cosmic abacus, where "good" (or wise) thoughts and actions rack up positive karma and future happiness and "bad" (or unwise) thoughts and actions rack up negative karma and future suffering. In other words, our patterns of thought and action perpetuate themselves.

For instance, when I was socially avoidant (scared of people), there would be occasions when I was invited out, to coffee with old friends let's say. Part of me would want to go. All of me would struggle with what to say, how to handle this. *Should I go? I should go. I want to go. I don't want to go. What's the worst that could happen? What if I embarrass myself? What if they think I'm fat? I am fat. I'm so stupid for being fat. What if they are super successful and happy and they see that I'm a total fuck up? Why does my stomach feel like I swallowed an anchor? Oh God, I'm nauseous. I think I'm getting sick; I can't go.* "So sorry, but I have to decline."

Ah, sweet relief. My face and shoulders relax a

little. The knot in my stomach is gone. I can stop pacing. Reward! Staying home triggered a good feeling. Now, next time I'm invited out, I'm even more likely not to go.

So, our habits create actions that perpetuate our habits. Metaphysically, *samskara* create *karma* that deepen the *samskara*. Physically, this is mirrored in neuronal pathways in the brain. Genetics and experience lay out connections in the brain and every time we reinforce our habits, the connections get stronger. I once had a therapist who described it with mashed potatoes and gravy. When you ladle gravy onto mashed potatoes, it begins to form channels to flow down. The more gravy that's ladled on, the deeper those channels become.

Practicing self-observation uncovers our *samskara*, our deep habits of thought. By slowing down enough to ask *What am I doing and why am I doing it?* we start to expose our motivations. It can be illuminating to approach self-observation without expectations and assumptions. A brief example: I had an aversion to adding things to my food and drink. If there was a special creamer available for coffee, I wouldn't try it. I avoided making sauces for which I didn't always have the ingredients in the pantry. I figured I did this because I was afraid I wouldn't like the new taste and adding whatever it was would ruin my food or drink. But after watching myself for a while, I realized that wasn't the case. I also wouldn't add veggie meatballs to spaghetti or walnuts to chocolate chip cookies. It wasn't because I thought I wouldn't like it; it was because I thought I would. And if I liked it with the new ingredient, I could never, ever make it the old way anymore.

Irrational? You betcha. And that's the point, once I knew my motivation and could see it was irrational, it became possible to face up to it and take action against it. We cannot challenge what we don't know exists.

The key to self-observation is mindfulness. Becoming aware of our thoughts, motivations, and actions means we have to be present. If you have started working with progressive relaxation or breathing exercises, you have started practicing mindfulness. Staying in the present can be hard work. We are used to dwelling in the past, worrying about the future, or distracting ourselves. We spend a lot of our day moving through routines, coasting on automatic. Training the mind to come back to the present is key. It also takes a fair amount of energy and effort. And that is why we need to pull over, take a break, ease up as much as we can when it comes to worldly activities, so we can devote ourselves to this inner work.

Also, at this initial stage we are not trying to change anything. Self-observation and self-acceptance go hand in hand. When you make a discovery, whether you like it or not, try to respond with *Oh, look at that.* Perhaps adding *That explains a lot.* My Kriya Yoga teacher says that one of the best responses to our own thoughts is "How interesting."

In the bigger picture, recognizing *samskara* is just the first step. Eventually, through acceptance and understanding, habits lose their hold over us. Through self-discipline, we burn through our accumulated *karma* and dismantle the very framework on which these habits are hung. The goal is to rid ourselves of all *samskara*, so we can live spontaneously from our Sacred center.

Koshas

It's almost time to talk about getting on the mat. First, let's spend a minute with the "self" part of self-observation. You may have had the sense from day to day or morning to night or hour to hour that the self is not a singular thing. We express this when we say "Part of me wants to do this," or "Part of me knows better," and the like. This is an important realization. The self, even when it's working well, is not homogenous. And when we experience anxiety, the variations in points of view, emotions, and preferences can feel like the world's most nauseating rollercoaster.

Besides navigating the rickety theme park rides of the mind, there are still more complications around the question, what is the self? Take these statements for example: I look good in black; I feel all right today; I didn't like that show; I'm learning Spanish; I got the job. Each of these refers to a different aspect of an individual: the body, emotions, likes and dislikes, cognition, and the self we present to others. A long time ago, before yoga was called yoga, the writer of the *Taittiriya-Upanishad* addressed this seeming schism in a model called the *panca-kosha*, or the five sheaths. The sheaths are layers of the self, like an onion or our planet.

Each layer carries the descriptive words *maya-kosha*. *Maya*, in this case, means appearance and reminds us that each *kosha* is only relatively real. Every part of the self with a small "s" is changeable and temporary. *Kosha* means sheath or casing but is often translated as "body," probably because most of us relate "casing" to sausages. Below are the five bodies and a brief definition of each.

1. *anna-maya-kosha*. Literally translates as the food appearance sheath. This is the material body, the physical form.

2. *prana-maya-kosha*. We've seen that word *prana* before. The second layer is the energy or subtle body.

3. *mano-maya-kosha*. This is what we usually mean when we refer to ourselves. Incoming sensory information, emotions, and preferences swim in this pool. It's often called the lower mind.

4. *vijnana-maya-kosha*. Variously translated as the intellect, understanding, and higher cognition. This is where discernment takes place. Plus, probably geometry and stuff like that. It's often called the higher mind.

5. *ananda-maya-kosha.* Any time you see *ananda* that means good times. The word indicates cosmic bliss.

It's from the ancient Indian texts called the *Upanishads* that we get the concept of each of us being a part of the Sacred whole. The terminology they used was *atman* and *Brahman* (only, there are no capital letters in Sanskrit so that's an English construct at work right there). *Atman* is the Spirit each of us has inside us. *Brahman* is the Sacred, the Absolute. And they are identical. *Tat tvam asi*; that art thou. And that is what is hiding at the center of the tootsie pop of your *koshas*; *ananda-maya-kosha* is the Self within all our other selves through which we participate in the universal dance of the Sacred.

Our job is to become aware of and sensitive to each of these layers of our being, to be able to start to observe and accept. We've already begun by relaxing the physical form, the food body, and engaging with the energy body through *pranayama*. The physical practice of yoga, the *asana* to which we turn in the next chapter, brings us into dialogue with each of the *koshas*. Through practice, it soon becomes apparent that the *koshas*, like the stages of growth, are not discreet units but that they weave in and out of one another, engaging, provoking, calming, and at times harmonizing with one another.

5

ON THE MAT

In this section we will cover reasons why the physical part of yoga is important, hesitations that may come up if you have never done *asana* (yoga postures) before, and I'll give some advice on how to navigate the wild and wooly world of yoga styles to find the type that's right for you.

As I mentioned in chapter one, it took me three years from deciding to try yoga to actually walking into a class. I had images of being surrounded by pixies—incredibly fit little women who knew exactly what they were doing and moved into every pose with grace and ease, two things I had not felt for a long time. My physique is more farm wife than pixie. People use adjectives like sturdy and good stock to describe me. It's better than plain old fat, which is what I figured I was for a long time.

Anyway, I was insecure about my body and I had

mental insecurities, too. I was afraid of not knowing what was going on, of drawing attention to myself and looking stupid. I was afraid I wouldn't be able to hear. I was afraid I would do things the wrong way and I had no tolerance for being wrong. I had no sense of competence. *What if I panic? What if I cry? Forget it. I'm not going.*

I had that conversation with myself every few months. In the meantime I read books and got DVDs on yoga. I practiced the DVDs until I had them memorized. I tried different styles. Some immediately resonated and some were immediately turned off. I was aware in an intuitional way that slow yoga was best for me. As much as I wanted to be able not just to do it all, but to master it all, faster styles of yoga didn't leave me feeling better the way slow styles did. More on that in a minute.

After I started on anti-anxiety medication and after I finally got hearing aids, I roped my sister into coming to yoga class with me. (She didn't really mind.) We lived in a small town and went to the only class I could find information about online. It wasn't the best but I didn't know that then. I liked it. I talked to the teacher after a few weeks about my anxiety (she had it, too) and my feeling that slower might be better for me. She referred me to an Iyengar teacher and the class that got me hooked.

You're Doing it Wrong: Yoga for Perfectionists

Danger Will Robinson!! As yoga has become more mainstream, it has also become more likely to perpetuate our cultural neuroses. The old standby to see this at work is the model on the cover of *Yoga Journal*: always skinny, always flexible, always happy, wearing designer gear, perfect hair, and just enough makeup to look like she doesn't need any. That's what sells their magazine, the promise that yoga will provide the cultural standard of beauty.

My favorite model of a yogi has always been Shiva, Lord of yoga, God of destruction and transformation. The proto-yogi, he sits on the peak of Mount Kailash, wearing equanimity, ashes, and a tiger skin. His dread locks are piled on his head and there is a cobra wrapped around his neck with its hood extended (a symbol of alert stillness). There's some cover art for you!

My point is it's easy to let yoga add to our anxiety instead of ease it. The wrong kind of class can breed competition and exacerbate perfectionism. We already have enough self-judgment and criticism. The best yoga classes undo the superficial cultural hang-ups that create anxiety. They foster self-acceptance, gratitude, and compassion toward self and others.

Self-Acceptance

Practicing yoga postures *is* practicing self-acceptance. Every time we step on the mat, we are there to practice being present, to witness and accept what we see with compassion and gratitude. We are there to practice contentment with what is without striving or struggling. We are there to practice letting go and trusting the practice. Changes will come and though they may not be the changes we expected or wanted, they are the ones we need.

You cannot be at peace if you're at war with your body. I have yet to meet anyone who didn't wish there was something different about the body in which they were living. Whether it's tight hamstrings, more weight than we might want, residual pain from an old injury, or some other perceived imperfection, everybody has something.

In the *Yoga Sutras*, Patanjali defines the perfect body as beautiful, graceful, and robust. We practice the physical postures (*asana*) of yoga to keep the body healthy so we can let go of concerns about the body and move on to greater concerns, like inner peace and spiritual liberation.

It isn't just the body that needs acceptance, the mind does, too. In any yoga practice it's easy to come up against frustrations, particularly in a class that moves too fast or is at the wrong level. It's also possible to find ourselves judgmental of self or of others. The process is the same: witness, accept, and let it go. *Oh look, I'm being critical. Time to move on.* Eventually, we hope to take these practices of self-acceptance and letting go off the mat and into our lives at large.

How to Know Where to Go

There are many different styles of yoga. The physical practices of yoga fall under the heading of Hatha Yoga. Hatha Yoga is a wide umbrella, covering *asana*, *pranayama*, *mantras*, *mudras*, and more. The tradition began in medieval India as an outgrowth of Tantra Yoga. The major insight of Tantra is that if there is only one reality and it is Sacred, then everything in that reality must be Sacred, too. Hatha Yoga focuses the work of coming into contact with the ever-present Sacred on the physical form.

The yoga-splosion of the last two decades has made choosing a beginning yoga class appear more complicated than trigonometry to an English major. But I am going to trim that mess back for you. People with anxiety need slow yoga. By slow yoga, I mean a style that eases into postures, holds them for a number of breaths, and eases back out of postures. So anything fast or hot is out.

To be sure, we do need cardiovascular exercise, too. There's nothing like a long bike ride or brisk walk to burn off the extra cortisol and adrenaline floating around in the blood stream. We just need to keep that separate from our yoga.

Before I list watch words for the more cardiovascular types of yoga, let me be clear that I am not saying there is anything wrong with these styles. They just are not the best for people who (a) already have the chemical cocktail of anxiety-producing hormones and neurotransmitters loose in their system and (b) are looking to slow down and become introspective.

Types of yoga that are usually heat building or done in a heated environment include Ashtanga (aka Ashtanga-Vinyasa), Baptiste, Bikram, Forrest, Moksha, and anything calling itself hot yoga. Power yoga and vinyasa (aka vinyasa flow or just flow) are descendants of Ashtanga. In vinyasa, you can expect a series of postures linked together, moving on both the inhale and the exhale with occasional longer holds. These are the types of yoga most popular in gyms. In fact, hot and fast yoga appear to be the most popular across the country. Or maybe they're just the most advertised.

There are many types of yoga where we can find a slower pace. Ananda, Intregral, Iyengar, Kripalu, Kriya, Sivananda, Svaroopa, and Viniyoga are all good choices for a beginner. More important than the style is the teacher. Many studios have teacher bios available online. I would recommend someone with significant experience, not just in yoga but in life. Yes, I'm saying go to someone older. Of course, you cannot know until you go if you are going to like a person's style of teaching.

I was extraordinarily lucky with my first Iyengar-trained teacher. Iyengar Yoga is known for being persnickety about alignment and their teachers have a reputation for being fierce task masters. I didn't know any of this when I showed up to class. This teacher was calm and soothing. Her concern for her students radiated. You could tell she was just delighted to be leading us through each and every meditative *savasana* (the relaxation pose at the end of class, pronounced shah-VAH-sah-nah). Done well, a yoga class is the most accepting, relaxing, and encouraging space in the world. It was in this class that I first heard the voice within (not the voice of my ego or conscience or any voice I'd heard before) say, "Yoga will save you."

Noticing my pursuit of a more spiritual experience, she recommended a teacher in nearby Bisbee, who was strongly influenced by Swami Satchidananda's Integral Yoga. Overtly spiritual in her language and presence and a master of spontaneous sequencing, I melted at some point in every Bisbee class. Tears in *savasana* became completely normal. Both classes became mainstays.

When I was ready to deepen my practice, both of these great teachers encouraged me to pursue teaching, too. That is how I came to Kriya Yoga. The Kriya tradition extends back through Paramhansa Yogananda. Concerned more with safety, comfort, and spiritual progress than with "doing it right," I feel privileged to be trained in this school and to now help train new teachers in this tradition.

My yoga journey has been one of happenstance and good fortune. That can happen in yoga if you let it.

10 Things for Anxious People to Know Before Going to Yoga

Below are a few tips for a person with anxiety who is going to a yoga class for the first or forty-seventh time. It may seem like a lot of information but the gist of it is to take care of yourself.

1. If possible, set up near a door, a corner, or a wall. Fewer people around means less sensory input. Less input means you are better able to focus on keeping your breathing calm and your attention turned inward.

2. Speaking of which, since yoga requires our attention to be turned inward, this means none of your classmates are interested in your abilities or lack thereof. As long as you don't disrupt their practice, they most likely won't even know you are there.

3. If you have an aversion to being touched, before class starts tell the teacher, "No adjustments, please."

4. If at any point you are asked to lie down on your back and this makes you uncomfortable, sit up. The basic movement of any pose or stretch done lying down can be done seated. Relaxation can also be done seated. If the teacher looks at you, smile. If the teacher asks if something is wrong, just say "Anxiety." A good teacher will understand.

5. If you are asked to close your eyes and this makes you uncomfortable, keep your eyes open and as relaxed as you can.

6. If you are asked to be face down, losing the ability to see around you and this makes you uncomfortable, bring yourself into a position where you can see without throwing your head back and chin forward. This action compresses the back of the neck and can cause damage if done repeatedly.

7. Keep backbends gentle. Bending back deeply squeezes your adrenal glands (on top of the kidneys), basically juicing them. The last thing we need when we're anxious is more adrenaline.

8. Yoga classes are meant to be places of self-acceptance and nurturing. If you don't get that vibe from a class or a teacher, don't go back to it. Try a different one.

9. If you become very uncomfortable and/or begin to panic in class, it's ok to take a break, go sit in the lobby, or even leave. The essence of *asana* practice is learning to take care of yourself. However, if you do leave a yoga class because of anxiety, try to go back as soon as you can. Don't let fear of fear keep you from such a valuable healing resource.

10. A sustained practice can provoke deep insights. Do what you can to accept these insights with compassion. Try not to ignore or bury them. Try

to sit with them and learn from them. Dealing with these insights is the real work of yoga.

Home Practice

Maybe you aren't ready to go to a yoga class. That's ok. Whether you are or whether you aren't, I strongly recommend having a home practice. Doing yoga at home lets you move at your own pace, deeply explore the poses you are attracted to, opt out of poses you don't like, and extend the relaxation before practice and the meditation after. It enables you to turn your attention completely inward for longer periods of self-observation. It is irreplaceable. But . . .

~ **I don't have room!** It doesn't take much room to do yoga. Most people have enough space between the couch and the TV. Just move the breakables.

~ **I don't have a mat!** Yogis, needless to say, haven't always had sticky mats. Traditionally, they sat on tiger or deer skins. In modern times, before the invention of the sticky mat in the 1980s, people used towels, carpet padding material, or gym pads. Point being, you don't need anything fancy to do yoga. Sticky mats are great but until you can get one, don't let that stop you.

~ **I don't have time!** Some of us can easily find half an hour by trading in some screen time, be it from the Internet, TV, video games, or whatever our distraction *du jour*. However, for many finding time is a legitimate concern. Time is a precious commodity. If you work and/or have children and/or are over-obligated, time can indeed be scarce. It can be challenging to make your own wellbeing a priority. Especially women are conditioned to find their own value in the value they hold for others. That is to say, we may give to feel our lives have meaning. And we think the more we give, the more meaning we have. It's easy for this to get out of control. Recognizing our intrinsic value can be a lengthy pursuit. For the time being, determine how much time you can reasonably commit and do it. Home practice sessions can be 20 minutes long, two days a week, and still produce fantastic results.

~ **I don't know what I'm doing!** That's ok. I'm going to provide a short sequence to get you started. Plus, if you are attending classes, you will quickly pick up stretches and poses that work well for your body. If you aren't going to classes, try getting DVDs (libraries have lots to choose from) or find teachers you like online.

Do's and Don'ts

Next are some guidelines for making the most of your home (or any) yoga practice.

Do enjoy your practice. This is a time to relax and

restore. Intention makes all the difference. Make a ritual of it by turning off your phone and lighting a candle or incense if you like. Set aside enough time and/or don't try to cram too many postures into the time you have. Consciously commit to being nurturing toward yourself.

Do take the time to turn inward before you begin. The mental aspect of yoga sets it apart from other types of exercise. Even before a short sequence, slow down. Either in *savasana* or in a seated posture try to be still for at least ten breaths or longer if you have the time and patience. Slowing down at the beginning of a practice makes our time on the mat more meditative. It also helps us generate movements from the inside out, in slow motion, which keeps us from overstretching or holding beyond our reasonable endurance.

Don't feel like you have to do every pose. Yoga should feel good and should never hurt. If you come across a posture that doesn't feel good, pass it by. You want to feel a stretch and to feel your muscles engaged, but there should never be pain or strain.

Do hold each pose for a few breaths. Flexibility takes time and patience. How long you should hold depends on your body and how you feel that day. Three to five slow, easy breaths is a good average to begin with. If your breath becomes fast or jagged, pause until it returns to a calmer rhythm.

Don't overdo. Pictures of poses are guidelines not

mandates. Remember that we practice yoga to enhance all the other aspects of our lives, not for the sake of yoga alone. Don't allow your practice to make you so tired or sore that you don't have the energy for the other parts of life.

Do *savasana*. Always. If you only have time for one posture, do *savasana*. Set a timer so you can let go completely. Take the time to settle in and relax. Then turn your attention to your breath. When your mind wanders, notice. Then let go of that line of thought and direct your attention back to your breath. It's normal for the mind to wander. Don't get discouraged. Your ability to stay with your breath will grow with time and practice.

Do enjoy your practice. Try to let go of your thoughts about the past or future and any judgments and just observe your body and mind as you move through each posture. Do what you can to keep your awareness not just inward but also downward. We spend a lot of time in our heads; during your yoga practice, try to keep your awareness throughout the rest of your body. That will help you to be fully present right here, right now, which is the only place and time we can truly be at peace.

20 - 30 Minute Yoga Sequence for Any Body

Here you'll find a well-rounded sequence of poses. It moves the spine through its many configurations; it cultivates strength, flexibility, and balance; and its primary components, mostly forward folds, soothe the nervous system. First, I'll explain the poses in detail, including modifications for people with physical limitations. Then I'll simply list the poses with illustrative stick figures, so you can see each posture at a glance. This series may take between 20 and 30 minutes, depending on how slowly you can let yourself move through the poses, the speed of your breathing, and how long you opt to stay in the beginning and ending relaxation postures.

If you don't have the patience for my explanations, skip ahead to the illustrations and come back to the instructions if you have questions. Most poses, besides the beginning and ending *savasana*, should be held or moved through for three to five breaths. A printable version of this and other sequences is available at yogatoeaseanxiety.com.

Corpse Pose (Savasana)

~ Begin lying on your back, legs extended toward the far corners of the mat. (I use "mat" for convenience. A towel, blanket, or just being on carpet is fine.)

~ Let your arms rest at about a 45 degree angle from your sides, palms face up.

~ Keep the back of your neck long and chin gently tucked in.

~ Relax. Using your timer, spend three to five minutes here, relaxing and watching your breath.

~ This is a great time to practice abdominal breathing or the four part breath. Begin to cultivate a slow, ease breathing rhythm to take with you through the whole practice.

Savasana modifications: If your lower back feels sore, stretched, or otherwise uncomfortable with your legs extended, bend your knees and place your feet just wider than your hips. Allow your knees to come together, so that your knees and inner thighs rest on each other. If your shoulders disagree with having the palms face up, place your palms face down or bend your elbows and rest your hands on your belly, middle fingers toward the navel. If your neck is uncomfortable, place a folded blanket under your head.

Pond mudra, aka full body stretch

~ After *savasana*, gently begin to stretch out your fingers and toes, then your arms and legs.

~ Bring your arms next to your head, reaching toward the wall behind you. Stretch from your finger tips to your heels.

~ This is called pond mudra because of the way the belly sinks down, creating a bowl or a pond. Even if your belly doesn't sink down very far (mine doesn't) try to feel the suggestion of the movement.

~ Tighten your whole body. Hold for a breath or two. Then relax. (It's like progressive relaxation only simultaneous instead of progressive.)

Pond mudra modification: If your shoulders are uncomfortable with your arms next to your head, extend them to form a "t" and stretch out from there.

Knee-to-chest pose

~ Bring your arms next to your sides and bend your knees. Place your feet on the mat.

~ Bring your knees in toward your chest and place your hands either behind your thighs on your shins. Hug your legs.

~ Rock from side to side, maybe even from elbow to elbow.

Reclined staff pose to Knee-to-chest pose

~ From knee-to-chest pose, extend your feet toward the ceiling and arms up past your head as they were in pond mudra.

~ Move with your breath. Exhale to knee-to-chest pose; inhale into reclined staff pose. Go back and forth three to five times.

~ Return your feet to the floor and arms next to your sides. Pause, relax, and breathe.

Transition to hands and knees

~ Roll onto one side, using your lower arm as a pillow. Slowly, press into the floor to rise up.

~ Shift to hands and knees.

Table pose

~ Bring your wrists under your shoulders and knees under your hips.

~ Spread your fingers wide and press into the balls of your hands and the pads of your fingers, so not all of the weight is on the heel of your hand.

~ Press the tops of your feet into the mat and pull your stomach in, so your navel moves toward your spine.

Table pose modifications: If your wrists hurt, you can pad under the heel to bring more weight onto the ball of your hand or come onto your forearms. If you have knee pain, try padding under your knees or do the pose standing using a chair, in which case you would stand facing the chair and place your hands on the chair seat. The next set of poses can be done from table with a chair.

Cat and cow poses

~ From table pose, on an exhale, curl your spine up toward the ceiling, as if you were rounding over a big beach ball. Let your head drop between your arms and tuck your tail bone. Your gaze should fall on your thighs or, for us bigger busted bodies, our cleavage. This is cat pose.

~ On your inhale, roll your pelvis in and slightly arch your back, coming into a gentle back bend. Keep your shoulders relaxed and away from your ears while you extend your neck long. Bring your gaze to center about two feet in front of your hands. This is cow pose.

~ Using your slow, easy breath as a guide, move back and forth between these two poses three to five times.

~ Return to table pose.

Downward facing dog

~ From table pose, curl your toes under. Press down through your hands and the balls of your feet while you lift your knees and hips. Press back through your arms so your hips go up and back while your legs unfold. Let your head come between your arms.

~ Keep your knees slightly bent, or bent a lot, to avoid over-stretching your hamstrings (the muscles on the back of the thigh). You want to feel a stretch, not a strain.

Downward dog modifications: If you have uncontrolled high or low blood pressure or eye problems where bringing your head below your heart is not recommended, you can do down dog using the wall. Facing a wall and standing about three feet back (depending on height and body proportions), bend forward enough to bring your hands to the wall at about shoulder height. With your head between your arms, stretch your hips back. Voila!

Forward fold

~ From downward facing dog, bend your knees and walk your hands and feet toward each other.

~ When your weight is balanced over your legs, come into forward fold.

~ Bring your hands to opposite elbows.

~ Let your head and neck relax. Hang out here for three to five breaths or as long as it feels good.

Forward fold modifications: Keep your knees as bent as much as you need to avoid overstretching your hamstrings. Forward fold is not recommended for people with uncontrolled blood pressure issues or eye problems where bringing the head below the heart may cause pressure in the eye.

Chair pose

~ From forward fold, with slightly bent knees, bring your hands to your thighs and rise up half way, so your back is relatively flat and parallel to the floor.

~ To come into chair pose either bring your hands together in front of the heart in *anjali* (aka *namaste*) mudra or, for a stronger variation, extend your arms next to your head.

~ Come up and back, as if you were sitting in an imaginary chair.

~ Hold for one to three breaths.

Mountain pose

~ Rise up and stand tall.

~ Think about bringing your stomach gently inward and your tailbone down. Lift your chest and roll your shoulders back.

~ Let your arms, shoulders, and face be relaxed.

~ Have some weight in the balls of your feet as well as in your heels.

~ Maintain this pose for five full rounds of breath.

Crescent moon pose

~ From mountain pose, lift both hands above your head. Wrap the fingers of your left hand around your right wrist.

~ Extend upwards through the right side of your body.

~ Side bend toward the left, stretching the right side of your body.

~ Hold for one to five breaths.

~ Repeat on the left side.

Stork pose

~ Start in mountain pose. Fix your gaze on a point on the floor.

~ With your hands together in *anjali* mudra, shift your weight over your left leg. Stand up tall.

~ Pick up your right foot and bring your knee up in front of you until it is even with your hip.

~ At this point, you may extend your left arm up toward the sky and right arm down toward the earth.

~ Hold for one to five breaths.

~ Repeat, standing on your right leg.

Stork pose modifications: If your balance is not cooperating, for this pose and the next place a hand on a wall or sturdy piece of furniture. If your knee doesn't come up even with your hip, it's no big deal.

Gentle dancer pose: aka quad stretch

~ In mountain pose, fix your gaze at a point on the floor.

~ Fold one leg back, bringing your foot up toward your butt.

~ Using either one or both hands or a strap or belt (or tie or sock or whatever), hold the raised foot.

~ To find more stretch, press your knee toward the floor and the hip of the raised leg forward.

~ Hold for one to five breaths.

~ Repeat on the second side.

Transition to floor

~ Return through **forward fold** to **downward facing dog**, holding each for a few breaths.

~ Lower your knees, coming into **table pose**.

~ Shift your hips toward your heels, walk your hands in toward your legs, and swing your legs around in front of you.

~ Slowly lower onto your back. Stretch out into **pond mudra** for a few breaths and then relax.

Bent knee twist

~ Bend your knees and bring your feet to the mat.

~ Extend your arms in a "t" shape.

~ Press into your feet and shift your hips a few inches to the right. Set your hips down and bring your legs close together. (You will feel crooked. It's temporary. Shifting the hips before twisting helps the twist to be better aligned.)

~ On an exhale, enter the twist by releasing your legs to the left and coming onto your left hip.

~ Find a comfortable position, allowing your legs to rest. You may bring a blanket or pillow under your left leg if it doesn't quite make it to the floor.

~ Maintain this twist for at least five breaths.

~ Roll onto your back. Shift your hips to center. Take a breath.

~ Repeat on second side.

Knee-to-chest

~ When you've finished the twist, bring your knees toward your chest.

~ Rock from side to side if that feels good.

Savasana

~ Relax in *savasana* for at least five minutes. Use your timer, so you can release completely.

~ Take time to settle in, scan your body for tension and soften as much as you can.

~ Your breath once again becomes the object of meditation. When your mind wanders, notice and practice letting go of those thoughts. Return your attention to the breath as many times as it wanders away.

~ After the timer sounds, gently and slow move your fingers and toes, arms and legs. Bend your knees and bring your feet to the mat. Roll to one side and press up to sit. This is a nice time to meditate, if and/or when that becomes part of your practice.

Stick Figure Yoga

Corpse Pose (Savasana), 3 to 5 minutes

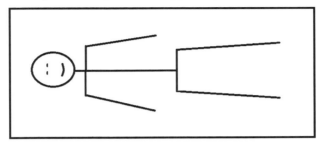

Pond mudra, aka full body stretch

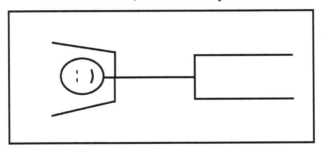

Knee-to-chest pose, rock side to side

Reclined staff pose to knee-to-chest pose, move
back and forth 3+ times

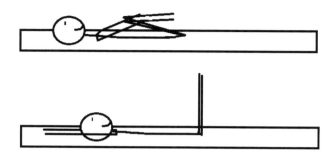

Table pose

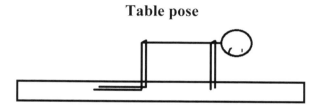

Cat and cow poses, move back and forth 3+ times

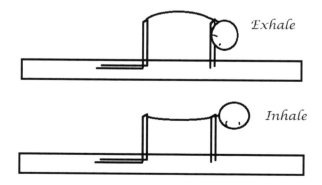

Downward facing dog

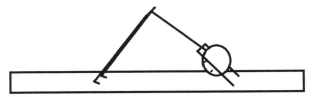

Forward fold

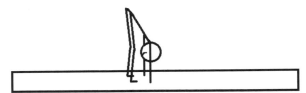

Chair pose

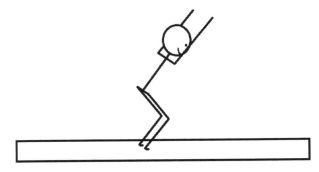

Mountain pose

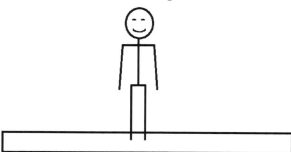

Crescent moon pose, both sides

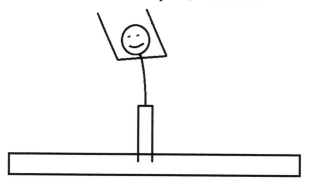

Stork pose, both sides

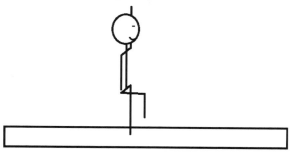

Gentle dancer pose, aka quad stretch, both sides

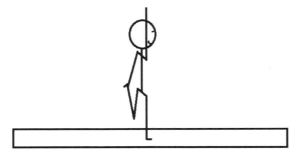

Bent knee twist, both sides

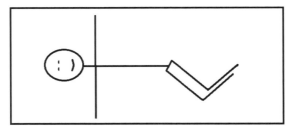

Knee-to-chest, rock side to side

Savasana, 5+ minutes

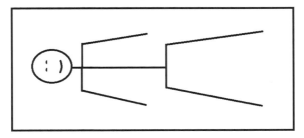

How Asana Practice Eases Stress

It's pretty widespread knowledge that practicing yoga helps relieve stress, but how does it work? Well, it's because of what we practice along with the postures: we practice slowing down and turning inward; we practice being physically relaxed; and we practice moving our attention from between our ears to elsewhere in our bodies. Being in class or guiding ourselves through a sequence gives us a break from our thoughts, not by producing a distraction but by pulling us into the present.

Yoga poses also help us practice staying relaxed in minorly stressful positions, like twists, or positions well outside our comfort zone, like inversions. We learn to pair a relaxed response to a stressful stimulus. In time, hopefully we can take that skill with us into crowds, traffic, tests, public speaking, or anywhere we would rather not react with fear.

The Road So Far

Part One: Yoga for Relaxation explored techniques we can use to slow down, shift our awareness from up in the head to down in the body, and release physical tension. No small feat. In Part Two: Yoga for Self-Acceptance we have learned about the stages of psycho-spiritual development (self-observation, self-acceptance, self-understanding, self-discipline, self-actualization, self-transcendence, and self-transformation) and the *koshas* (food body, energy body, lower mind, higher mind, and bliss body). And then we covered some basic yoga postures.

Focusing on the body and the breath (the first two *koshas*) is the doorway to change. It is our initial training in self-observation, self-acceptance, and self-understanding. It is even the beginning of self-discipline. Focusing on the body leads to insight into the mind. In Part Three: Yoga for Fearlessness, we are going to move from observation of the mind being a byproduct to being the central act.

PART THREE

YOGA FOR
FEARLESSNESS

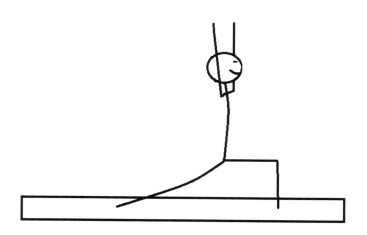

6

THINGS NOT TO DO

In yoga nothing is ever simply prescriptive. Every piece of advice, every suggested perspective is practical. And so it is with Patanjali's *Yoga Sutras*. It is a practical guide to Self-realization.

Search for books at amazon.com using the key words "Yoga Sutras" and you will get 4,215 results. On Google, "Yoga Sutras" returns 1,570,000 hits. There is a lot out there on the *Yoga Sutras*, so much that my rebellious side spent a good while searching for a different way to present the information in these two chapters. *The Sutras*, that hoity little voice in my head said, *have been done to death.* Well, it turns out there's a reason for the popularity of this old, terse set of aphorisms. They are good at what they set out to do.

What we know about its author, Patanjali, can fit in the next three sentences. He probably lived in the second century CE. He was certainly an authority, probably the leader of a sect or school. And he appears to have compiled these ideas rather than invented them, gathering all the current knowledge of yoga in one place. That's it. That's all we know, historically.

Mythologically, though, there is more. According to Feuerstein, "Hindu tradition has it that Patanjali was an incarnation of Ananta, or Shesha, the thousand-headed ruler of the serpent race that is thought to guard the hidden treasures of the earth. The name Patanjali is said to have been given to Ananta because he desired to teach Yoga on earth and fell (*pat*) from Heaven onto the palm (*anjali*) of a virtuous woman, named Gonika." (2001, 214). He is often pictured as having the upper body and head of a man and the lower half of a coiled snake.

The Yoga Sutras is a collection of 195 or 196 (depending on the source) concise statements. Each one of these aphorisms was meant to be given due consideration, unwoven and pondered, studied, discussed, and expounded upon by a teacher. Unfortunately, there are no commentaries in existence from the second century CE. The oldest commentary, *The Yoga-Bhashya* by Vyasa, dates from the fifth century CE. So, what those of Patanjali's time would have learned from their guru as they worked through the *Sutras* is largely a matter of speculation.

Textual analysis has shown that *The Yoga Sutras* is actually a redaction or compilation of ideas from two different schools of yoga: *Kriya* Yoga and *Ashtanga*

Yoga. The *klesha* that we talked about in chapter one (remember them?) come from the *Kriya* Yoga portion. For these two chapters, I will use *Ashtanga* (Eight-limb) Yoga as a framework for our discussion. (This *Ashtanga* Yoga is different from, and about 1800 years older than, the *Ashtanga-Vinyasa* style of Hatha Yoga mentioned in chapter four.)

The Eight Limbs

The eight limbs of *Ashtanga* Yoga are as follows: restraints (*yama*), observances (*niyama*), posture (*asana*), breathing exercises (*pranayama*), sense withdrawal (*pratyahara*), concentration (*dharana*), meditation (*dhyana*), and ecstasy (*samadhi*). This chapter and the next will be devoted to the restraints and observances, of which there are five each. The other limbs will be covered after that.

First, a brief reminder of why we practice in the first place. The problem is suffering, life is full of it. Suffering is caused by the *klesha* (wrong knowledge, I-am-ness, attachments, aversions, and clinging to life). The way to end suffering is to compassionately detach from our attachments and aversions until we can serenely deal with life's curve balls. With that comes fearlessness, the ability to remain at peace regardless of the vicissitudes of life. (If this seems familiar that's because it's a quick summary of the discussion of *klesha* in chapter two.) The eight limbs are Patanjali's advice on *how* to practice in order to bring about that equanimity.

The restraints (*yama*) and observances (*niyama*) are guidelines to help us create and keep harmony in our lives. They are similar to the morals advocated by all widespread religions; only the reasoning behind them is not to go to heaven, avoid damnation, or even to keep our communities running on an even keel. Instead, their whole purpose is to allow our minds to quiet down. Following these precepts helps us keep our energy centered and not scattered. There is less to worry about when our actions are not undermining our objectives.

The eight limbs build upon each other. The restraints and observances start to quiet the mind, preparing it for the later stages of meditation. The restraints (*yama*) are nonharming (*ahimsa*), non-lying or truthfulness (*satya*), non-stealing (*asteya*), chastity (*brahmacharya*), and non-greed (*aparigraha*). The observances (*niyama*) are cleanliness or purity (*shaucha*), contentment (*samtosha*), austerities (*tapas*), study (*svadhyaya*), and devotion or surrender to a higher power (*Ishvara-pranidhana*). Each one has something to teach us.

Non-harming/Ahimsa

Imagine you are talking to a good friend, one of your favorite people. This is someone for whom you care and have deep respect. This person tells you they're suffering. How do you feel? What do you want to do?

Do you want to comfort them? Help them? Or do you berate them for not having the wherewithal to get their shit together? For being weak and wearing their heart on their sleeve? Of course you want to comfort them, because you, like most people, are not a complete jerk.

Unfortunately, it's normal for many of us to be jerks to ourselves. The practice of non-harming is much easier when it comes to how we treat others. As we practice self-observation, the harshness of our self-judgments can be stunning. The first step is to witness. Some things I've called myself: *a total mess, dumbshit, fucking idiot.* Things I used to say often: *Jesus, Amy, you do this all the damn time. Get over it. Snap out of it. Grow up. You should be better by now.* Ah, the foul-mouthed, condescending jerk that lives in my brain. What an ass! I would never talk to anyone else like that. Why is it ok to talk to myself like that? It isn't.

A word needs to be said here about "should." Perfectionism, achievement needs, worry, obsession— these all lead to telling ourselves a lot of shoulds and shouldn'ts. *You should be happier. You should stop picking at it. You shouldn't need a break yet.* And on and on. Now, I am not in the camp with those who think we should never use the word "should." First of all, there are things we should do. For instance, we should brush our teeth. We should take the best care of ourselves that we can. Getting rid of a word is too simplistic and leads to just replacing "should" with another word: *You ought to get more done. It's stupid to be afraid.* Instead, we need to look at each instance. Determine if the demand is reasonable or unreasonable, kind or callous. Usually, the place to start is in distinguishing the difference between needs and wants. Sure, I wish I had a great attitude about doing the house cleaning and the laundry and the shopping all on the same day, but telling myself *You should be happy* isn't going to change the fact that I hate it. What I *need* to do is get my chores done. Being happy about it doesn't really matter.

Allowing ourselves to express the full range of emotions is important. We're human; emotions are part of the deal. Trying to be cheerful or stoic or whatever all the time isn't going to fly. We get angry, we get sad, we get disgusted. The key is to feel it, entirely. Watch the emotion, where it sits in the body, how it moves through. Every emotion is a wave. Witness the wave. It will help you feel more in control. It will help you become more empathic. And it will help you befriend your emotions, instead of letting them build into scary, overwhelming meltdowns.

Non-harming goes hand in hand with compassion and forms the foundation for all of the other restraints and observances.

Truthfulness/Satya

"I'm fine." That's the lie I've told the most in my life, to myself and others. I remember telling a therapist that I was a "high-functioning agoraphobe." That doesn't even make sense! But we want to be well and we will tell ourselves we are, that what we feel and think is normal. Everybody worries, everybody wants to succeed, everybody has rituals. Even if that were true, who cares what everybody else does? What do you *want* to do? How do you *want* to be in the world?

I'm not saying we should never say "I'm fine," or that we should run around telling everyone who asks "How are you today?" about our challenges. But tell your family. Tell your friends. You need their support. Everybody needs to ask for help sometimes. Let other people help you, especially in this period of being pulled over. The stigma you may perceive around anxiety is just a perception. What we think about what other people think is usually wrong; it's based on our own harsh self-judgments. We can't know what other people think unless we ask them. And after we ask, we have to learn to take people at their word and not read into it. Unless their sarcasm is five hundred decibels louder than their words, accept what people say at face value. No more *He's just saying that to be nice*, or *She didn't really mean it*. Experiment with letting other people take responsibility for saying what they mean.

Truthfulness as a rule, as a standard by which to live, helps us function more smoothly. Lies are hard to keep track of. Lies haunt us and come back to bite us. If you feel you have to lie to keep a person in your life, perhaps it's best to let that person go. Non-harming precedes truthfulness for good reason. There may be times when a lie could prevent harm. These cases are rare and need to be approached with caution and discernment. For the most part, telling the truth may be difficult, but in the long run it's the way to go.

There's more to truthfulness than just not lying. There's letting truth shape your life. To do this, you first have to know the truth by which you want to live. This is a central aspect of self-identity. What is your truth? I'll tell you mine: love gives meaning to life and peace is worth seeking. I didn't come by this easily.

If you've ever entered therapy, you may have been asked, "How do you see your ideal day?" When I started in recovery, my ideal day was detailed. I woke up before everyone else, took a shower, and had a healthy breakfast. I was calm and even-handed wrestling my kid into his school day. I spent the morning getting work done and on and on. Like I said, detailed. A few years into the process, I had to find a new therapist. When he asked "How do you see your ideal day?" my answer surprised me. "Really," I said, "I just want to wake up at peace." As the words came out of my mouth, I knew they represented a deep truth. Something relaxed at the core of my being with that epiphany. Since then, peace has become a central motif in my healing.

No one can tell you what your guiding truth should be. It may even change along the way. That's ok. Find the truth that works for you today. And tomorrow, find the truth that works best for you tomorrow.

Non-Stealing/Asteya

Most of us figured out that stealing is unwise a long time ago. First, as toddlers we learned that supremely difficult lesson: "mine" and "not mine." We learned taking "not mine" would lead to trouble. Some people get stuck right here: stealing is bad because it leads to punishment. Others go on to recognize that not taking "not mine" is a sign of respect for others.

Taking objects that do not belong to us clutters our lives with guilt, shame, and possibly more concrete consequences. So does taking on less tangible things that also are not ours. Taking on responsibilities that are not meant to be ours is a common problem for those of us with anxiety. I worried about everyone. No, I worried *for* everyone, even though nobody needed me to. I worried about what my husband would eat, what he would wear, what mood he would be in when he got home. When he had a headache I thought it was my fault. When we were invited out to dinner, I worried about how I could make it so everyone there could be comfortable and have a pleasant time. I even worried about people I didn't know. I worried what the checkout girl thought of my groceries. I worried what the people driving down the street thought about how my dog pulled me along on our walks. (See earlier quote from RuPaul, "What other people think of me is none of my damn business!")

Really, nobody cares, strangers especially. Unless you are helping someone to or inhibiting someone from getting their needs met, you are most likely not even on their radar. As for close family and friends, being a worry-wart isn't only unnecessary, it can be annoying, aggravating, and for kids, stunting. Mostly though, it doesn't hurt anyone but the worrier. It can be a real load off to recognize the difference between "mine" and "not mine" when it comes to responsibilities.

Switching tracks but staying on the topic of stealing: anxiety steals. In my experience, it starts by taking self-confidence and filling us instead with "what-ifs." Given time, it takes any sense of control, of humor, of balance. It empties us of joy until there's nothing left, until you can stare into the darkness and not be afraid because *anything* would be better than this. I have a very clear memory of taking the garbage out one night and just standing in the carport, wishing I could dig my fingers into my sternum and crack my ribs open like a cabinet. Then, covered with gore and with my heart exposed, maybe people would see on the outside how much pain I felt on the inside. Anxiety steals our very lives away from us.

When my son was getting to the age where he needed me to take him to things like birthday parties and swimming lessons, things that terrified me and triggered panic, I knew I had to get help so he could lead some semblance of a normal life. I probably should have before. Instead I let him spend his first few years with a jack-in-the-box for a mom—never knowing when I would pop or whether I'd be angry or desperately sad when I did. I deprived him and his dad of years of stable family life. I deprived myself of years of being able to relax, play, laugh wholeheartedly, love unselfconsciously.

Anxiety is not fair. No one asks for it and it isn't anybody's fault. It just happens given the right genetic predisposition and the wrong circumstances. But by not taking care of it, not getting the help I needed, I wasn't just hurting myself. It's scary to get help and change is hard. Therapy and prescriptions, if you need to go that route, can be expensive, especially without insurance. There are other first steps you can take, community groups and online forums can be tremendously supportive. Just reading books, unfortunately, does not cut it. We need the help and support of other human beings.

There are only so many days in this lifetime, only so many breaths each one of us will breathe. Appeasing anxiety instead of overcoming it robs you and your loved ones of that precious, potentially joyful time.

Chastity/Brahmacharya

Brahmacharya used to mean celibacy. Here's how it used to be and still is in some traditional families in India: according to the 2000 year old *Laws of Manu*, there are four stages of life. First, the student stage lasts until young adulthood. Next, in the householder stage, a man (this is all about men, remember we're talking 2000 years ago) works and raises a family. Thirdly, in the forest dwelling stage, after his first grandchild is born he can retire to the edges of the community, figuratively and literally. And finally in the ascetic stage he renounces his old life, to include all relations and even his name, and becomes a wandering mendicant in search of spiritual freedom.

Of course there have always been those who could not wait for old age to follow the spiritual path. Whether young or old, if a person chooses to live as a renouncer (*sannyasin*), celibacy follows. Sex creates attachments, to say nothing of offspring! For a wandering mendicant who seeks to be free of worldly ways, celibacy makes perfect sense. But for us, we need a different approach.

Chastity, at its most basic, implies not getting it on with just anybody. Sex can make fledgling relationships really complicated really fast. And since the point of these restraints (*yama*) is to establish a mindscape as free from intrusive fluctuations as we possibly can, the best sex is that based in intimacy and commitment. Especially if you are just beginning to work on your inner self, now is not the time to start a new physical relationship. Let that be part of being pulled over. If it's meant to be, it'll be there when you get back on track.

Possibly even more so than with sex itself, our thinking can become preoccupied with being sex-y. As we all know because we live it every day, our economy is based on consumerism, consumerism is based on marketing, and marketing is based on exploiting our insecurities. Simply by virtue of being awake, we are pummeled with messages questioning if we are thin enough or fit enough. Is your skin smooth enough? Are your eyelashes long enough? Are your blemishes covered? Is there hair anywhere but on your head, where it needs to be luxuriant and smooth? The beauty industry would love to make sure we don't leave the house without everything from our toenails to our eyebrows done to their dictation. And since all of the markers of beauty, at least for women, add up to a skinny, buxom, prepubescent seventeen year old, no one ever meets the mark.

No wonder the U.S. has the highest rates of plastic surgery and body dysmorphia. No wonder we have weird headlines like "Sexy at Sixty." At sixty, I hope to exude a lot of things—confidence, compassion, wisdom—but sexy? Here is another societal norm we must overcome to be healthy. It's normal to want to feel attractive. It's crippling to accept that there is only one definition of what is attractive and to base our opinions of ourselves on an impossible standard.

While we're on the topic of externally decreed standards, let's talk about diets. Diets are miserable for people with anxiety. They take over every second of the day, creep into every decision and every nook and cranny of mindspace. Most importantly, being on a diet separates us further from our bodies. Instead of being an integrated whole of body-mind-spirit, the mind is pitted against the body, trying to dictate what the body should want and what it can and cannot have. Yes, it's important to eat nutritious food. Yes, it's important to take care of health issues when they arise. If your weight is not a health issue, experiment with not letting it be an issue at all. We cannot be at peace if we are at war with our bodies.

Sex can be a chance to relax completely, spontaneously giving and receiving affection and love with the most important person in your life. Or sex can trigger our deepest insecurities. Approaching our own sexuality with compassion and detachment is a first step toward embracing this sacred act.

Non-greed/Aparigraha

Want want want. In the grip of anxiety, there's a lot to want. By turns I would want to live somewhere else, to have a different job, a different house, a different body, a different brain. I wanted to be a different person. I wanted people to want less from me. When generalized anxiety strikes, we look for a cause. Even if we know that cause is free-floating cortisol and adrenaline, the first stressor that comes to mind usually gets the blame. If we could just fix *that*, whatever that is this time around, we would feel better.

My fallback when I was overwhelmed was to plan a vacation. I wanted to be somewhere else, with no responsibilities and none of the people that I knew. I would plunge into online hotels sites and reviews of things to do in whatever my target area was. For a few hours or even days, it would provide an escape. Then the worries would set in. *Vacations are expensive. What if it's crowded? Will we drive or fly? Which one is worse? Who would we impose on to take care of the animals? Should we get someone to watch the house? What if someone breaks in while we're gone? There probably won't be any vegan restaurants. We'll have to eat mostly in the room. Should we bring food or buy it there? Will we have to do laundry? I hate having to do laundry in hotels.* And just like that, I added vacation to the list of things I wished were different.

Our culture of materialism feeds on this discontent, this wish that things were different. Marketers aim advertising right at us and tell us their products will give us peace of mind and take away our stress. Once your house is impeccably furnished, you will be able to relax. Once you get that new car, traffic will disappear. Save time! Save money! Make yourself or someone else happy! All by buying stuff. Even if it isn't outright advertising, we need to be aware of whether the movies and shows we watch, the books we read, the magazines we scan in the checkout line, any media we let into our heads are sowing discontent in us.

The paradox is that to create change we have to accept things the way they are. I'm not saying we have to *embrace* the way things are today, just that we need to be realistic about where we are right now. Observe what is actually going on and live with it, without trying to ignore it or pretend it doesn't exist. For small moments, practice simply letting everything be as it is.

When we have thoughts we wish were different, thoughts we wish we didn't have, we need to be realistic about the fact that they exist, but that doesn't mean we have to allow them to continue. In cognitive psychology, the effort to discontinue a thought is called "thought stopping." I've met some sensitive souls who aren't comfortable telling themselves to "stop." They think that's too harsh. If you're in that camp, find another term that works for you. When you see a thought that is irrational, harmful, or pessimistic *pause.* Recognize it. Say to yourself, *That isn't helpful.* Or *That isn't reasonable.* Whatever makes the most sense to you is what you need to use. The vital idea here is that you *do* have control over your thoughts. You *can* change your thoughts. I find it helpful to tell other people my most asinine thoughts. Saying them out loud creates perspective and makes those thoughts easier to stop the next time around. And there will be a next time around. The goal is to make it so these types of thoughts become less and less frequent.

We've been talking about acceptance throughout these pages. This *yama*, non-greed, is one more opportunity to see acceptance from a different angle. All the *yama* are things we ought not to do: don't be mean, don't lie, don't steal, don't sleep around, and don't be greedy. And they can all be phrased as things we ought to do, too: be compassionate, be truthful, take only what is yours, honor your sexuality, and accept what is.

7

THINGS TO DO

While the *yama* (restraints) were originally intended to be things we should not do, the *niyama* (observances) are things we *should* do. Keep in mind that all of this is practical rather than prescriptive advice. Patanjali recorded a tradition that says if you want to still the mind, follow these steps. By attending to these suggestions, there is less mental chatter and we become more settled, better able to let go of regrets about the past or worries about the future and be at peace, right now.

Purity/Shaucha

Usually interpreted as purity or cleanliness, *shaucha* can also mean "to cry with tears," possibly because of the cleansing tears provide. Back in the days when Patanjali was writing, physical cleanliness was less frequent and more important, what with the general grubbiness and unsanitary conditions of life before plumbing. Long life has always been important to yogis, because that means longer to work toward liberation. And yogis, perhaps due in part to this hygienic advice, were known to live extraordinarily long lives.

These days physical cleanliness is pretty standard, leaving us free to explore the deeper meaning of this observance which is purity of thought. Mentally, we are more cluttered than ever. There is constant input and outflow. And to escape the onslaught, instead of quieting down we switch channels, find something different to read or listen to. In other words, we increase the input. We have cluttered houses, cluttered calendars, and cluttered minds.

Part of self-observation is taking a realistic look at what we own and how we spend our time. Which of our possessions are really valuable, in that they actually add value to our lives? Do we have stuff that weighs us down? Clutter in the spaces where we spend our time creates completely unnecessary stress. Letting go of that which you no longer need on the material level is liberating and can make it easier to let go of that which you no longer need on the emotional and mental levels as well.

Another useful exercise is creating a map of your day to see how you really spend your time. This can be a list or something more freeform. For one average day keep track of what you do and how you spend your attention. It doesn't need to be in excruciating detail. It's just an experiment to see if there are ways you might be able to unclutter your time.

There is a deeper discussion of purity here, of purifying the mind to more fully reflect Reality. This is why we practice. We are polishing the mirror so that the little self may become transparent and the Sacred can shine through. We will talk more about this later.

Contentment/Samtosha

Samtosha (contentment) is the flip side of *aparigraha* (non-greed). In order to not want things to be different than they are, we must work at accepting what is. How can we be content in a world where so much is so out of whack? In our own lives and more widely, there is suffering. Are we supposed to ignore that? No. Contentment is not about sitting back in a recliner and putting your feet up with a sigh, although that's nice to do sometimes. Contentment is about accepting this moment, exactly as it is.

We should work for change, each in the way that calls to us. It's called *loka samgraha*, which translates as "drawing together of the world" (Feuerstein 2008, 191). In essence, we align ourselves with the Sacred in order to better function as part of and contribute to the welfare of the world. Another paradox: to help others, we must first work on ourselves. To move down the path, we must learn to stand still.

Allowing this moment to be just as it is, without

needing to judge it as good or bad, without needing to criticize or approve—that is contentment. And contentment is hard. Again, we are going against a lifetime of cultural training. From our first breath we are taught some things are good and some are bad. The more we grow the more we are indoctrinated into this either/or mentality. Nothing just is. It is always named and categorized according to its qualities or uses. Experiencing an event without judging it can be like trying to see a word without reading it.

One tool that can help increase the likelihood of moments of contentment is gratitude. Taking a few minutes a day to come up with things that are going well, things for which we are grateful, increases our capacity for empathy and optimism. Moments of contentment are all we are looking for right now. As we grow, perhaps we will learn to recognize the world with all its blemishes as an expression of the Sacred and to see decisions as wise or unwise instead of good and bad. For now, let contentment be a place to rest.

Self-discipline/Tapas

The literal translation of *tapas* is "heat." Before there were yogis, in the ancient-ancient sacred texts called the *Vedas*, people who performed austerities were called *tapasvin*. One of these austerities, still performed by yogis today, was *panch-agni-tapasya*, the five-fire-austerity. In this ritual, four fires are lit, one in each direction, and the yogi meditates in the center of them, beneath the fifth fire of the sweltering Indian sun. Talk about *heat*.

An austerity is a self-inflicted hardship. Some more familiar austerities might be fasting or abstinence or silence. There are several reasons to perform austerities. They can break us from routine, alter our consciousness, and remind us of higher aims. Feuerstein referred to self-discipline as "creative self-frustration" (2003). In other words, we must create situations that take us beyond where we are comfortable and force us to grow.

Self-discipline sounds daunting, but it is only through changing our actions that we can change our habits of mind. And there is no reason to believe we have to start big and go even bigger. Small changes can be just as important when it comes to generating transformation. Committing to a discipline that you know would be doable, such as practicing a breathing exercise for five minutes a day, is a perfectly legitimate form of *tapas*.

One extremely frustrating form of self-discipline I engaged in, as I mentioned earlier, was making a list of public activities that scared me and doing one a week until I'd done them all. It's a trite cliché but "feel the fear and do it anyway" has proven good advice. Once we do what we fear and live through it, it's easier (not *easy*, but easier) to do the next time and the next.

Beware! For those of us prone to obsession, self-discipline can get out of hand. When committing to a practice, be reasonable. After the initial "pulled over" phase, do your best to establish balance between caring for yourself and other responsibilities.

When I started yoga, I treated it like everything else I've ever taken on; it was just another thing to be conquered, to be mastered, as quickly as possible. I wanted to be the most flexible. I wanted to be the most knowledgeable. There's an old article from *The Onion* titled "Monk Gloats over Yoga Championship," where the winner shouts, "I am the serenest!" I wanted to be the serenest!

There are a lot of different definitions of yoga and competition doesn't appear in any of them. What a relief it was to finally let go of the need to be the best at yoga. Then I could *enjoy* the practice, tune in more fully to my body and breath, stop struggling with my thoughts and just let them flow by. Another paradox: releasing the need to be good at yoga makes us better at it.

As well as being a *niyama,* self-discipline is the fourth stage of psycho-spiritual growth. The stages, to recap, are self-observation, self-acceptance, self-understanding, self-discipline, self-actualization, self-transcendence, and self-transformation. As you may have discovered for yourself, these are not discrete steps. Even to begin self-observation takes a little discipline. And the rewards from self-acceptance and self-understanding make self-discipline more likely to be maintained or even deepened. The stages create an interdependent cycle that loops back on itself, jumps forward sometimes, becomes a knotted mess sometimes, and eventually weaves together the fabric of our spiritual lives.

Self-study/Svadhyaya

Translating as "one's own study," *svadhyaya* refers to both the study of one's self and to studying, traditionally, the ancient sacred texts. Self-observation is obviously part of self-study. So is self-understanding. Knowing why we think and act the way we do is essential. Do other members of your family, either biologically or otherwise, have mood disorders? My family tree is festooned with crazy. But DNA isn't the only way to inherit anxiety. Emotions and thinking patterns are contagious. We learn how to react to the world by watching those around us. For many of us, as children we already had a biological predisposition toward creating more anxiety-related chemicals or fewer calming chemicals, and then the people in our lives either weren't equipped to help us deal or exacerbated our anxiety with their own. The idea is not to place blame but to recognize the pattern so we can better understand and transcend.

Not all mood disorders are hereditary. Many different types of events can create deeply rooted anxiety. Have you lived through a traumatic incident or multiple traumas? Have you experienced great loss or chronic insecurity when it comes to basic needs like food, shelter, and love? Did important people in your life have unreasonable expectations of you or none at all? Unfortunately, there are probably miles of questions we can add to this list.

My favorite line from Patanjali's *Yoga Sutras* is this: "What is to be overcome is future sorrow." Understanding the origins of our behaviors can be illuminating. The important thing is not to get hung up here. Causes are in the past. We are concerned with the present and preventing "future sorrow."

On the subject of self-study, two quotations come to mind: one from a bumper sticker, "Don't believe everything you think," and the second from Albert Einstein, "Problems cannot be solved at the same level of awareness that created them." One of the most frustrating parts of anxiety was that I did not know which voice in my head to trust. For example, being invited to meet up with extended family for a weekend getaway would provoke a flood of voices. The voice of anxiety would say, *I don't want to go. What if I get lost? What if they think I'm ridiculous?* The voice of the tyrant said, *Don't be stupid, just go.* The voice of the parent, *It'll be good for you to go.* The voice of the child, *You can't make me. I'm going to stay home under the covers.* The saint said, *I will go and make the world a better place for everyone.* The rebel said, *Fuck that noise, I'm staying home and getting drunk.* The queen demanded, *I will go but only if I can have my own room and leave whenever I want.* The pirate goes, *Aahr matey, yer walkin the plank fer sher.*

Ok, there is no pirate voice in my head on a usual basis, but you get the point. Which voice should I listen to? I didn't know, until one evening in an Iyengar-based class (slow pace, long holds), I was in Triangle pose. I don't remember feeling especially serene or anything special. I was just there and a voice in my head that I'd never heard before said, "Yoga will save you." I believed it completely. There was no question in my mind that this voice spoke the truth.

Now, when the cacophony of competing voices starts up, I know the best thing I can do is not listen to any of them but just stop. Decide not to decide. For real, I set the timer for five minutes and just sit on the couch. I don't try to meditate; I don't try to do anything. I just sit and breathe. And more often than not, I find I've cleared a path for that voice of truth to be heard. Sometimes right away, sometimes later that day or the next. For me, finding this voice, what I consider to be my true voice, has been the greatest gift of self-study.

This observance has never been just about introspection. Reading and studying important books falls under *svadhyaya*, too. This includes any book that helps you grow as a person. Books about anxiety and positive psychology, books about spirituality from any tradition, books about people who inspire you; it's all "one's own study." Be selective about what you put in your brain and what you choose to believe. Fill your mind with thoughts and stories that make your mind a better place to live.

Two of the aspects of Eastern paths I've always admired are their experimental nature and the recognition that different personalities have different spiritual needs. Taken together, what this means is that when you come across a suggestion, evaluate it. If it's attractive to you, try it out and see if it works for you. Keep in mind, though, that the suggestions that are the most repellant to us may just be the ones we need the most.

Devotion/Ishvara-pranidhana

Ishavara means Lord and *pranidhana* means surrender to or devotion to. Together they mean devotion to the Lord. *Ishvara* also refers to the Sacred that dwells within each of us, as they are One and the same. Many of us can benefit from devotion to an external personification of the Sacred, a Lord. Which Lord? Remember that the yogic tradition comes from India, where there are many gods and goddesses. Remember, too, that in this worldview All is One. There is one fundamental consciousness underlying, permeating, and containing all creation. This is variously called Brahman, Purusha, God, the Universe, Reality, and the Sacred among other things. Goddesses and gods are recognized as anthropomorphic figures that make the Sacred easier to relate to for humans. The god or goddess we choose to worship is our *Ishta-devata*.

Some people squelch at the idea of submitting to a higher power. I did. It didn't seem rational. Where's the proof? I didn't want to be duped and look stupid. I had faith in the process of yoga because I had experienced it. But faith in something bigger, something all-encompassing, was hard to come by.

As a child I was brought up to believe in a God who was an old white man in the sky. If someone had explained to me as a young teenager that God doesn't look like that, that God doesn't have a gender, and that we made up that picture so we could relate to the idea of God, maybe I wouldn't have turned so completely away from the religion of my family and my ancestors. But nobody did. And when I started having spiritual experiences—feeling like I was part of a Whole, intuitions of calling and a sense of expansiveness—the flying bearded guy was nowhere to be seen.

Faith is a choice. *Ishavara-pranidhana* asks no more than that we recognize a force that is other than our small selves. The Sacred we are asked to revere is already a part of us and we are part of it. It is simply the life force and energy residing everywhere, always. Any other attributes you want to give it are up to you. The concept of choosing your god or goddess might seem utterly foreign to those of us brought up in a monotheistic religion, where there is no God but God. That hasn't changed; the Sacred is eternal and unchanging, regardless of what we call it, but the face we ascribe to it? That's just another part of our mental experience. You don't have to give it a face at all. It has been useful to me to consciously decide which goddess or god best suits my spiritual goals and devote myself to keeping that form in mind.

My view of devotion may seem pragmatic and existential and that's what works for me. You have to come up with what works for you. Faith is worth cultivating. Having a standard to live up to helps us know when we're on the right path. It also makes the world feel like a friendlier place and lets those of us who take on the weight of the world surrender some of that burden.

Summing Up

The reasoning behind the *yama* and *niyama* is to get our inner lives in order so that we can stop questioning and second-guessing ourselves and put the cares of the world aside. It's no easy feat, and we cannot wait until this work is done before we move on or we would never move on. Each of these precepts will continue to be a part of the path. Non-harming, truthfulness, non-stealing, chastity, non-greed, purity, contentment, self-discipline, self-study, and devotion—all continue to evolve and deepen in significance until they are no longer rules we take on from the outside in but they become spontaneously generated principles that flow from the understanding and experience that we are all part of one Sacred existence.

8

MEDITATION

One way to organize our thoughts about our path so far is to look at it as if we've been working our way inward through the *koshas*. The outermost sheath is food body. This is the focus of progressive relaxation and the physical practice of yoga. Next, the energy body is what we work with through breathing exercises. The next two layers, the lower and higher minds, are targeted in the self-observation, self-acceptance, and self-understanding that we practice through the *yama* (restraints) and *niyama* (observances). What's left is the the bliss body.

As we start talking about steps further along the path—self-actualization, self-transcendence, and self-transformation—if these seem super far away, like you're looking at them through the wrong end of a telescope, don't worry about it. It's a map. When we start on a trip, we need to trace out the whole route so we know where to turn and how many peanut butter sandwiches to pack. While it may take some time to make progress down the path, it's motivating to know that we're headed toward a place where we can let go of the fear that if we stop holding it together it will all fall apart; a place where we can feel peace and joy; a place of unconditional acceptance and love.

Meditation

Everybody recommends meditation. It can be an absolute life saver. Research on meditation began in the 1920s and really picked up speed in the 1970s. Physically, meditation has been shown to lower blood pressure, improve sleep, alleviate gastrointestinal problems, and help people cope with pain. It's been shown to improve focus, memory, cognitive flexibility, creativity, empathy, and compassion. Therapists use it to help treat depression, anxiety, obsessive-compulsive disorder, substance abuse, and eating disorders. But, as I mentioned earlier, from the depths of anxiety and/or depression, meditation blows. "Oh, your thoughts are your enemy? Just sit still. Clear your mind." What kind of advice is that? I'd rather chew tin foil.

You're doing it wrong. You're wasting your time. This isn't going to help. Did you turn the stove off? Where are the cats? This is dumb. Nothing will help you. Relax. Shut up. Did I put that appointment on the calendar? How much time has passed? Ad infinitum. That was meditation on a good day. A bad day was when there was some event to cling to, some decision to be made, some real or imagined interpersonal slight to hash over. Clear my mind? Yeah, right.

It wasn't until I figured out that meditation isn't something you can choose to do that I learned how to sit. Let's go back to the eight limbs for a minute because the last three are the answer.

The first two limbs are the *yama* and *niyama*. Next come posture (*asana*) and breathing exercises (*pranayama*). (Historical side note: When Patanjali wrote the *Yoga Sutras*, *asana* just meant meditation posture. It wasn't until Hatha Yoga was born around the tenth century CE that *asana* came to mean the yoga postures like those we know and love and sometimes tolerate.) The fifth limb is called *pratyahara*; this means sense withdrawal, turning inward. It's an effect of *pranayama* and the first step toward a new, peaceful state of consciousness.

The last three limbs are concentration, meditation, and bliss or ecstasy (*dharana*, *dhyana*, and *samadhi*). Together these three create the process of *samyama*. In modern parlance, when people say "meditation," they usually mean this process of *samyama*. Thing is, of these three states, only concentration is something you can choose to do. Let me explain.

When we first begin to "meditate," we need something on which to concentrate—a candle flame, a word, our bones, our breath. In concentration, we focus our attention on an object, allowing that object to completely fill our mindspace. When our attention drifts and thoughts come up, as will happen, we are to gently but firmly come back to the object of concentration. Attention and concentration are like muscles in that they can be built up through exercise.

This is the first step, and in a bit I will lead you through just such an exercise. But first a few words are in order about sitting to "meditate."

How to Sit

First of all, during this type of practice we need to be relaxed and alert. If the relaxation part is difficult, try sitting after progressive relaxation. If the alert part is difficult, and you find yourself falling asleep, try it at a different time of day. We all go through cycles during the day when we are more sluggish or more energetic.

If you haven't moved your body much for a while before sitting to meditate, take a minute to stretch. Do some side bends, some twists, and a few seated cat-cow stretches. I like forward folds to stretch out my spine before I stack up my vertebrae.

When you sit, sit tall. Keep the back of your neck long; this will make your chin tuck a little and direct your gaze slightly downward. It doesn't matter if you sit on the floor or in a chair. However, if you are on the floor and your knees are high or the lumbar curve in your lower back disappears, put a folded blanket under your hips to bring your spine into a more neutral position. You'll be able to sit longer that way. If your back gets tired, use the chair back or sit against a wall.

Your meditative seat should be comfortable. If, during the practice, part of your body starts to tingle or cramp or even just feel slightly uncomfortable, change your position. Turning your senses inward is a prerequisite that can only happen if the body is comfortable. The physical practice of postures (*asana*) helps build the necessary strength and flexibility to sit for longer periods.

Practice: Visualization Concentration

Read through all the directions before you start, not least because step five is to close your eyes.

~ Choose an object that is calming to you. Maybe a candle flame, a polished stone, or a simple picture.

~ Arrange yourself so you are seated with the object about two feet in front of you, so it is in your line of sight when you sit tall.

~ Set your timer for three to five minutes and start it.

~ Look at your object. Study it.

~ Close your eyes and visualize the object. Recreate as many details in the visualization as you can.

~ When the image fades and cannot be brought back to mind, open your eyes and study the object again.

~   Continue studying the object and visualizing the image in turns until the timer chimes.

~   Then, set aside any attempt to think about anything in particular. Just relax for a minute.

That's it! Every other type of concentration and/or meditation builds on this simple practice. You can use a short prayer, a word, or some other auditory stimulus instead of a visual one and that becomes *mantra* meditation. However, make sure it's an idea with which you want to fill your mind.

There is a popular practice of breathing in something positive (like peace or relaxation) and breathing out something negative (like fear or frustration) but by repeating to yourself that which you want to get rid of, you are filling your mind with a negative just as much as with a positive. If you want to practice like this, breathe in what you want to build (e.g., serenity) and breathe out what you want to give (e.g., compassion).

A more advanced type of meditation uses the breath itself as the object of concentration, without trying to change it. It's harder because the breath is so subtle; there is less on which to focus and keep the mind occupied.

Deeper States

This is important: meditation is something that happens while you're practicing concentration. Meditation is a state of consciousness in which you don't have to work at holding the object in mind. It's just there. Concentration takes effort, the constant return of your attention to your object. Meditation is effortless, the barrage of other thoughts has quietly ceased. Only you and the object exist in your consciousness during meditation. You make concentration happen; meditation happens to you. At first, meditation lasts for brief and fleeting moments. The residual effect is tranquility.

Samadhi is an even deeper state of absorption into the object of concentration and meditation. It has been described as union. I have only ever been to the outskirts of *samadhi,* and from those ephemeral glimpses I've brought back joy, absolute unbridled joy. When this happens my heart is so full I want to jump around and weep at the same time. It is more than a peak experience, more than everything just seeming right and feeling good. Sensations are beyond crisp. Connections between everything are obvious. My heart and mind overflow with compassion. I feel like a live wire! The first time it happened, it scared the hell out of me. I was afraid it was a delusion. And, having lost touch with reality before, I was in no hurry to do it again. Fortunately for me, I have a teacher to whom I can turn, whom I trust. When I told her what had happened, she smiled and assured me I was not going crazy.

According to yoga, we have *samskara* or deep patterns of thought and behavior. These create *karma* or consequences which usually serve to deepen the *samskara*. In other words, we have habits that create actions that reinforce our habits. Touching *samadhi*, they say, burns away our *karma* and eventually dismantles our *samskara*. In other words, accessing our bliss body allows us to let go of our habits and change our brains' pathways. When the *samskara* are gone we are liberated. Then we are free to live spontaneously from our Sacred center. That's the goal, the treasure the maps lead to. It's so important, I'm going to say it again: When the *samskara* are gone we are liberated. Then we are free to live spontaneously from our Sacred center.

Up from the Bottom of the Barrel

I'm 40 now. For the most part, I'm better. I still pick, but not nearly as much. I still occasionally think people hate me for no reason, but only until I catch myself. I'm not in therapy anymore, but I see a psychiatrist every three months. Maybe I will always be prone to anxiety. I have to be ok with that. What matters is that I can feel joy now. I can play, laugh, love, and sit still.

I've moved from my small desert hometown to Tucson. Moving was rough. For a while, every single day held some new experience. But I like Tucson. I feel more freedom here.

I drive in traffic every day. I don't like it, but who does? I can handle it without sitting bolt upright and clenching my teeth. Just last week I navigated the one-ways of downtown, solo, and used metered parking for the first time in my life. I'm completely comfortable in drive-throughs, car washes, and parking garages now.

There are still things that trigger panic. The idea of having to travel out of state alone, for instance. Gah! Just the thought of it and my shoulders are tense. I have that hollow feeling in the pit of my stomach. I know I could handle it. But *what if I get lost? What if I miss my flight? What if I do something stupid? What if something bad happens to me? I've never rented a car before. What if, what if, what if?* I know that if I would just go, just do it a couple times, the fear would ease. *But it's so expensive. It would be selfish of me to travel just to get over a fear. I should wait until there's a good reason. Like I'm not a good reason!* The inner dialogue continues.

What I'm not afraid of anymore is being alone, feeling unloved, and losing the people I love. I'm not naïve enough to think I can't lose them, but I don't spend my time dreading it anymore. And, in one last paradoxical turn of events, by releasing my fear of losing those I love, I've learned to open my heart and let them and others more fully in. Life is so much sweeter now. Before, I shielded myself from rejection by not letting people know how much I cared. Now I can offer my compassion openly.

Recapitulation

The ideas I've written about here have given me my life

back. The understanding that we are more than this body, this ego, and this set of experiences is by turns humbling and liberating. I do what I can to remember that attachments and aversions are just habitual reactions to passing phenomena. It takes practice to overcome the *klesha*: lack of knowledge, I-am-ness, attachments, aversions, and the will to live. But the rewards are entirely worth it.

I try to slow down, to remember to be mindful and to observe and accept my thoughts. I remember coming across Feuerstein's seven stages of psycho-spiritual growth for the first time (self-observation, self-acceptance, self-understanding, self-discipline, self-actualization, self-transcendence, and self-transformation). It was like hearing about gravity or the laws of motion for the first time as a child. Part of my mind said, *Well, yeah. Of course that's how it is*, as if it should be intuitively obvious to everyone. And another part was utterly mystified at the simplicity and beauty and perfection of it. The same is true for the *koshas* (food body [*anna-maya-kosha*], energy body [*prana-maya-kosha*], lower-mind [*mano-maya-kosha*], higher-mind [*vijnana-maya-kosha*], and bliss body [*ananda-maya-kosha*]). Pure genius!

I first learned about the eight limbs of Patanjali's *Yoga Sutras* in college, where they unfortunately had little effect on me. I memorized them, spit them out in essay form, and promptly forgot about them for a dozen years. Now, they're part of my everyday life (restraints

[yama], observances [niyama], posture [asana], breathing exercises [pranayama], sense withdrawal [pratyahara], concentration [dharana], meditation [dhyana], and ecstatic union [samadhi]).

These three models—the seven stages, the *koshas*, and the eight limbs—are all maps of the same terrain.

Slowing down through postures and breathing exercises opens the door to self-observation and self-acceptance of the food body and energy body. Examining the motivations of our lower and higher minds through the restraints and observances furthers self-understanding. Practicing self-discipline deepens our observations, acceptance, and understanding of all the *koshas* and cultivates self-actualization. *Samyama*, the three-fold practice of concentration, meditation, and *samadhi*, brings us to the bliss body and self-transcendence. Every step of the way is self-transforming.

Fare Well

Maybe it seems like there's a lot to do. Please, don't think you have to do everything I've recommended. It's too much all at once. Let's see, there's slowing down; pulling over; learning to relax your body; learning to control your breath; taking up a home *asana* practice and going to class; sustained introspection; journaling; evaluating your possessions; creating a map of your day; asking other people for help; practicing gratitude; and making a list of things that scare you and tackling those fears.

These are actions that have helped me over a number of years. They don't have to be done all at once. They don't even all have to be done. Try to see it as a list of possible self-improvement projects. The first step, the only one that might be considered mandatory, is learning to control your breath. Just do that, then see what follows. Pick a new self-improvement project when you're ready. Don't overload yourself and don't quit!

Yoga means different things to different people. I hope for you it can come to mean relief from anxiety and peace of mind. Nothing temporary can hurt you. You are Eternal. There is nothing to fear.

Works Cited

David, Martha, Elizabeth Robbins Eshelman, and Matthew Mckay. *The Relaxation and Stress Reduction Workbook.* 6th Ed. Oakland, CA: New Harbinger, 2008. Print.

Feuerstein, Georg. *The Encyclopedia of Yoga and Tantra.* Boston: Shambhala, 2011. Print.

---. *The Lost Teachings of Yoga.* Boulder, CO: Sounds True, 2003. CD.

---. *The Yoga Tradition: Its History, Literature, Philosophy and Practice.* 3rd Ed. Prescott, AZ: Hohm Press, 2008. Print.

Seligman, Martin. *What You Can Change and What You Can't: The Complete Guide to Successful Self-Improvement.* New York: Knopf, 1993. Print.

Tulku, Tarthang. *Openness Mind.* Emeryville, CA: Dharma Publishing, 1978. Print.

Index

abdominal breathing, 33-37, 70

ahimsa (see non-harming)

ananda-maya-kosha (see bliss body)

anna-maya-kosha (see food body)

anxiety, v, 14-15, 22, 24, 25, 41, 63, 93, 96, 97, 100; hereditary, 51, 110; environmental, 42-43, 45, 110-111

aparigraha (see non-greed)

asana (see postures)

Ashtanga Yoga, 88-89

Ashtanga-Vinyasa , 61, 89

asmita (see I-am-ness)

asteya (see non-stealing)

atman, 55

attachments, 19-21, 89, 125

austerities, 90, 107-108

aversions, 20-21, 89, 125

avidya (see ignorance)

bliss body, 55, 85, 116, 123, 126

brahmacharya (see chastity)

Brahman, 17, 18, 55, 113

breathing exercises, 10, 32-39, 52, 55, 89, 118, 126

celibacy, 97-98

chastity, 90, 97-100

clinging to life, 20, 89

compassion, v, 16-17, 20-21, 45, 49, 58, 59, 89, 92, 117

competition, 58, 109

concentration, 89, 118-122, 126

contentment, 59, 106-107

detachment, 16-17, 20-21, 45

devotion, 90, 113-115

dharana (see concentration)

dhyana (see meditation)

ego , 17-19, 47

eight limbs, 89, 90, 118, 125-126

Einstein, Albert, 111

emotions, 45, 53-54, 92, 110

energy body, 54, 55, 116, 126

faith, 114-115

faster styles of yoga, 61

fear, 14-16, 20-21, 24, 41-42, 108

fearlessness, 16, 89

Feuerstein, Georg, 4, 43, 88, 108

five fires austerity, 107

food body, 54, 55, 116, 125, 126

four stages of life, 97-98

God, 114

gods and goddesses, 113, 114

gratitude, 58, 107, 126

Hatha Yoga, 60

higher mind, 54, 116, 126

home posture practice, 65-78

hot yoga, 61

ABOUT THE AUTHOR

Amy Vaughn has been studying Eastern philosophy and mysticism for over 20 years. She was drawn to Hatha Yoga as a means of managing a severe anxiety disorder. Her practice and teaching center on stilling the mind through self-acceptance and compassion.

Amy earned her 200 hour teacher training certificate from The Yoga Connection (Tucson, AZ) and an 800 hour certificate in the History. Literature, and Philosophy of Yoga through Georg and Brenda Feuerstein's Traditional Yoga Studies. She has a B.A. in Religious Studies and Psychology and an M.A. in Sustainable Communities.

Besides teaching gentle and traditional Hatha Yoga, Amy leads workshops on the history, philosophy, and practice of yoga and mentors teacher trainees. You can find her teaching classes around Tucson and online at DesertSkyYoga.com.